Working With Hearts

Unveiling the Cath Lab

Angela Sinachi

ISBN: 978-1-959392-28-6

Dedication

To the Almighty God, the giver of dreams.

To my parents and siblings, who taught me how to dream.

To my husband, for fanning those dreams to flames.

To my children, for keeping the dreams alive.

Acknowledgment

First and foremost, I would like to give all glory and praise to God Almighty for his unending waves of blessings upon me. I am also grateful to Chukwujekwu Sinachi, my number one fan, and husband, who has always been very supportive of me. Thank you for being an encouraging voice that urges me to take the next step. I remain eternally grateful.

To Mr. Michael Juma, my work brother. I totally appreciate your invaluable contributions. Thanks for allowing me to see through your eyes and patiently reading my numerous drafts. Thank you!

To my Cath lab family, Susie Hendry, Alberto Fernandez, Efraim Esponilla, Santhi Santhiyothin, and Hiep Tran. Thanks for critiquing, suggesting, and fine-tuning the ideas and stories; I appreciate it. To my ICU/ACU colleagues, I remain grateful.

I would also like to express my profound gratitude to the following cardiologists/interventionists who have been so supportive of me, especially those who took time out of their already overwhelming schedule to proofread and give valuable suggestions.

To Dr. Ryan Armstrong and Dr. Long Cao, you guys are amazing. You took your time to read my manuscript line upon line and, like college professors, graded the work and offered suggestions. It meant the world to me. Dr. Vijaiganesh Nagarajan, thanks for believing in me and constantly whipping up that hunger to learn with your incessant quizzes as we worked. That knowledge came in very handy. Thank you, Dr. Sachin Kumar Amruthlal Jain, for allowing me to glean a wealth of knowledge from your article on Takotsubo. To Dr. Karomibal Mejia, I appreciate your kind words of encouragement.

I am also grateful to my parents in the faith, Pastors Toye and Wumi Ademola, Pastors Wole and Bimpe Olowolayemo, Pastor Stephania Hicks, Rev. Veronica Ebie, and Mrs. Yvonne Jobe.

Contents

About the Author

Angela Sinachi, LLB, BL, BSN, RN, CVRN-BC, is a Certified Cardiac Vascular Registered Nurse. She holds a BSN from the University of Texas Health Science Center, Houston. She is a brilliant and compassionate acute care nurse with seven years of nursing experience. A lover of knowledge and literature with a background in Law. She hopes to educate her patients and the general public on what goes on in the Cath lab and how to better care for their hearts and general well-being.

Angela is happily married, and the union is blessed with four amazing children. She is involved in different organizations, helping abused women, troubled teenagers, and the less privileged.

About the Author

Preface

The heart is one of the most essential organs of the human body, and Cath lab professionals work with it every day. Heart attacks, heart failures, heart arrhythmias, and vascular diseases are just some of the emergencies seen in the Cath lab regularly.

Dealing with such a sensitive organ also brings with it a host of pressure and responsibility. When you essentially hold a person's life in your hands, you do all you can to keep them from slipping through your fingers. Often, this can take a physical and emotional toll on you.

When a heart patient enters the Cath lab, it's a race against time to protect them from the jaws of death and give them new life. *Working With Hearts* details all that goes on when you work with hearts, the kinds of emergencies these medical personnel witnesses, and how they deal with the trauma and scars that these cases leave behind. The stories are based on real-life experiences witnessed by my colleagues and I, written to help readers better care for their hearts.

Preface

Chapter 1
The Pager

beep* *beep

I heard something in the distance but couldn't really make out what it was. After a long day at work, I was finally getting some much-deserved rest for my exhausted body and mind. In my sleepy state, I didn't even stir at the familiar yet strange sound.

beep* *beep

There it was again. This time, however, my brain comprehended what it was. With eyes wide open, I immediately flung out of bed and picked up my pager from its usual place, my nightstand, and read the message: "Code STEMI. ER 3". A STEMI is the deadliest type of heart attack. It was time for war. I quickly got out of bed with my pager in hand, grabbed my keys and my battle gear (my scrubs), and ran out the door. In no time, I was on my way to the hospital, which was 20 minutes away from my house. I looked at my watch: 12:40 am. I had hardly slept, and yet I was anxious to arrive at the hospital to attend to the patient because it has been ingrained in me that the quicker a STEMI patient gets treated, the less damage occurs to their heart.

As I drove to my destination, I started thinking of ways to

treat the patient while considering all the possible complications that could arise. This was just another day in the life of a Cath lab team member or any other health care professional, where you never really know what to expect.

***

Everyone has a different purpose in life. Some want to become successful, some want to be famous, and others want to be rich. We all have different dreams or goals that motivate us and keep us moving forward. Of course, there is more to life than just selfish or self-centered goals, but we are so preoccupied in pursuit of those goals that we often lose sight of what truly matters. I believe the primary purpose of life is to be loving, giving, sacrificing, and being true to yourself.

Everyone seems to need a “bandage” to heal from different things, whether a physical wound, a broken heart, a bruised ego, or a scar from the past that refuses to heal. While some people can overcome their wounds or simply bury them deep inside, others choose a different path, one that allows them to benefit others and help them heal. Who are these people, one might ask? Anyone who contributes to the wellbeing of others - health care professionals, law enforcement officers, firefighters, clergies, and any other social welfare workers, to name a few. Without these people working for our health, safety, and security, the world would be a very different place.

I, too, am one who chose the path of helping others. Being a natural-born leader who is task-oriented, with a lot of confidence and great problem-solving skills, and a team player, I was always one to make quick decisions and take risks, sometimes based entirely on my intuition. Being sensitive, caring, and empathetic at the same time, I realized the field of health care was best suited for my skills and personality, and I found my true calling as a nurse. I work as a certified cardiovascular registered nurse (CVRN-BC) at the Cath Lab.

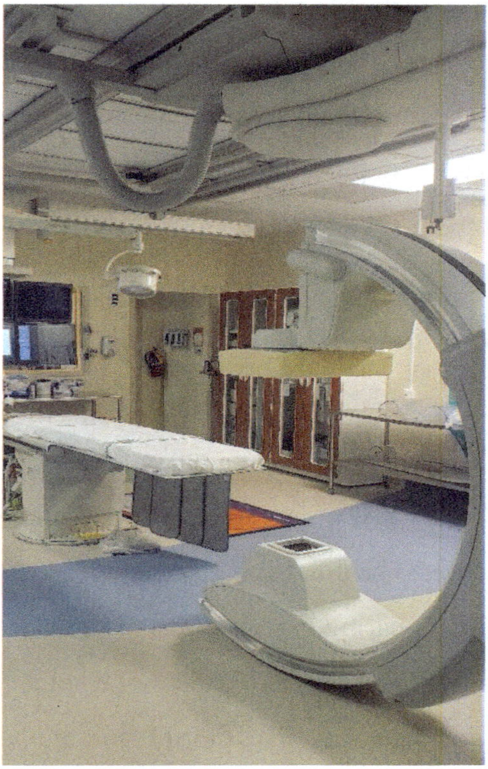

A standard Cath lab

What is a Cath lab, and what do we do there? A Cardiac Catheterization Laboratory, or Cath lab, is where tests and procedures such as angiogram, angioplasty, ablation, stent placement, and implantation of pacemakers or ICDs are done. Cardiac catheterizations are performed to diagnose and treat certain cardiovascular issues. Cath labs are equipped with special imaging equipment to analyze arteries and see how well they are working. They are staffed by a team of specialists. For a cardiac catheterization, the doctor puts a tiny and flexible hollow tube called a catheter into a blood vessel in the patient's arm or groin. They then direct it through the blood vessel into the aorta and heart. Once the catheter is in place, different tests can be conducted. For example, doctors insert a small amount of dye into the arteries and heart chambers through the catheter to check blood flow under running X-rays. This is also called a coronary angiogram.

Becoming a nurse has changed my perspective about people and life in general. When a patient comes in, they become your responsibility. You are entirely devoted to treating them and nursing them back to health. Living in this society, we have grown accustomed to only caring for ourselves or those we know. For us nurses, everyone is the same. Regardless of whether we know them or not, our patients are our first priority, and attending to them is of utmost importance.

Being a healthcare professional is to put your life on hold for the welfare of others. We are like soldiers, always prepared to fight because the pager is nothing less than a clarion call for battle. It sets off an alarm that awakens every fiber of our being, and once it goes off, we have no choice but to answer it and to do so promptly. No matter where we are, what we are doing, who we are with, or what time it is, we must abandon everything and rush to the hospital. It sometimes becomes quite difficult to maintain our personal and professional lives because there is no fixed time for our professional life and no telling when or how long our services might be required. Whenever we are needed, we must present ourselves. So, our profession takes over our lives, and our personal lives take a backseat.

We are so busy looking after our patients that we often miss out on different events and gatherings with friends and family. It all comes with the territory, missing out on birthdays, anniversaries, parent-teacher conferences, and your kids' games. When people are peacefully sleeping in their homes, we are working in the lab in the middle of the night and attending to an emergency. When people are enjoying their days off or spending time with their family on Christmas or Thanksgiving, we are either already at work or always expecting the pager to go off any minute. We never get the weekends or holidays off because health problems are not selective of days or holidays. Such is the nature of our job.

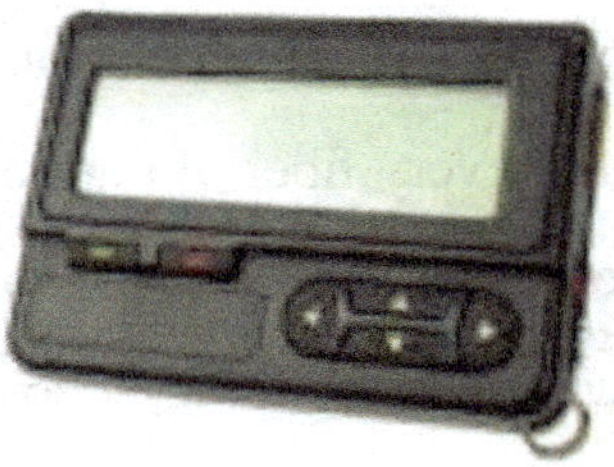

A standard pager

For healthcare professionals, our whole life revolves around our work. Even when there are no updates from the pager, there is always this thought in the back of our heads that it could go off any minute, especially in the middle of the night or in the wee hours of the morning. Whenever we are doing something, that thought always gnaws away at our minds. It sometimes feels like we are on house arrest because we are either at home for a short while or at work most of the time. Sometimes we just don't have time for anything else. We have to plan our personal life in a way that coincides with our professional life - no going to the beach, no going for a weekend trip somewhere with our family. Our life activities become restricted to a 30-minute radius from the hospital. Whatever we have to do, it must be done within this limit. Grocery shopping, going to the mall, meeting up with a friend, we can never be too far from the hospital because we never know when we might be needed.

Every time we hear the chime on our pager, we must abandon whatever we are doing and rush to save a life. Whether we are at a party, in the checkout line at a grocery store, in the middle of music practice, or simply cooking, we have to leave everything and answer that call.

So how can we just leave everything and get straight to work? What if we are in our night suits? Well, seeing doctors and other staff members report to the hospital in their night suits or loungewear is not uncommon. But it really doesn't matter what you are wearing as long as you show up. Since there is so much uncertainty in this line of work, you create a balance between your personal and professional life and learn to live life on the go. No matter where you go, you either wear your scrubs or keep them handy in a bag in the front seat or in the trunk of your car, ready to be put on for action.

Once you are in your scrubs, you become a completely different person. Your contact with the outside world is put on a temporary hold, and all you need to focus on is the work at hand.

Of course, the lab isn't continually undergoing an emergency, and we have slow days too, but when a case arrives, we are informed about it, and our presence is required at the earliest. At that moment, everything else goes straight out the window, and all we can only think about is the patient.

If you think about it, a pager essentially separates life from death. One missed message from a pager, one slight delay in responding to the message could mean death for someone. It isn't only our lives that revolve around this small device but also the lives of our patients. I have seen cases where someone slept through a page, which delayed a patient's care. In cases of heart-related problems, even the slightest of delays can be detrimental to the patient's health, sometimes even fatal.

Besides informing us about cases, the pager also keeps us updated about the patient's condition, allowing us to be prepared when we report for duty. When the alarm bell goes off, you suddenly get a jolt of energy, even if you are exhausted and haven't slept well in days because of the adrenaline rush. It opens up all your mental faculties. As you keep getting reports and updates on the patient's condition on your way to the hospital, you start preparing a mental care plan. *How long till I get there? What is the first thing I should do? What should be done next if the nurse has given the patient a particular medication?* Every possible scenario and procedure takes over your mind, and those thoughts invade your mind, not leaving room for anything else.

I keep referring to my work as war or a battlefield because it is just like that. We are in a constant battle every day, fighting to free our patients from death's clutches, refusing to let go. The fiercest battle of all is that of a Cath lab nurse treating an unstable STEMI patient.

STEMI stands for ST - Elevation Myocardial Infarction and is considered the most severe type of heart attack. A STEMI occurs when the heart does not get the oxygen-rich blood that it needs to function correctly due to complete or nearly total blockage of a coronary artery. Coronary arteries are blood vessels that supply the heart muscle with oxygen-rich blood that enables the heart to keep up with the task of supplying every part of the body with blood. Blockage in coronary arteries is typically caused by the process of arteriosclerosis. This is the hardening and narrowing of the coronaries due to plaque buildup. Plaque is made up of excess calcium and cholesterol deposits. If a plaque ruptures, a blood clot forms, and such clots further disrupt the flow of oxygen-rich blood in the arteries.

Arteriosclerosis can be triggered by both modifiable and non-modifiable risk factors. Modifiable risk factors include hypertension, high blood cholesterol, diabetes, obesity and overweight, smoking, and a sedentary lifestyle. Some of the non-modifiable factors are the patient's gender, genetics, and advanced age. According to CDC, men are more likely to have heart attacks than women.

A STEMI is usually detected by an electrocardiogram which is also known as an ECG or EKG. This is a quick, safe and painless test that records the heart's electrical activity. With the help of EKGs, doctors are able to check heart rhythms and diagnose a heart attack and poor blood flow to the muscles of the heart of a patient. An ECG consists of a PQRST complex. The ST region indicates when the heart is at rest. When a person has a heart attack, the ST segment becomes abnormally high above the baseline, i.e., unusually elevated. So, during a STEMI, the patient's ST wave increases.

Once the patient begins to experience chest pains and cannot be relieved by MONA (Morphine, Oxygen, Nitroglycerin, and Aspirin), or beta-blockers, it indicates that the blood vessels have not widened enough to get blood to the heart muscle. With each passing second, there is a risk of infarction or dead heart tissue.

While some patients choose to ignore the pain and ride it out, others can feel it immensely and describe the pain as "an elephant sitting on their chest." Some patients, such as those who are diabetic, may not feel severe pain due to diabetes-related nerve damage. For example, instead of feeling a pressure-like pain in their chest, they might feel discomfort in their arm or jaw or no pain at all. Whatever the case and regardless of whether the patient is in pain or not, every STEMI case is an emergency and is treated as such.

Damage from a STEMI is usually irreversible, and you can only keep it from worsening. If immediate reperfusion therapy is performed, significant damage can be avoided. However, without immediate reperfusion therapy, which is a medical treatment to restore blood flow through or around blocked arteries with drugs, procedure, or surgery, a STEMI patient can develop Q waves, which indicate the parts of the myocardium that are dead or scarred.

This is also why pagers are so important. Even a minute of delay can make the condition of a heart go from bad to worse, and sometimes a patient may never recover, that is, if they even survive. There are instances where patient care is delayed because someone slept through the call or could not get their car out of the driveway because it was blocked by someone else. Whatever the reason, there is no room for error when it comes to heart patients.

Although life and death are a part of our lives, and we see them repeatedly, losing a patient never gets easy. The most challenging cases are particularly those where a patient presents with very mild symptoms or no symptoms at all, but they are gone in the blink of an eye. Every patient you treat becomes like family, and losing a family member is never easy. It takes a heavy toll on you. Such cases leave a mark on us, but we have to go about our day as if it never happened because we have other patients to care for. With each patient we lose, our fight to save our future patients becomes stronger because we can't lose again. We give it all we have for our internal vindication.

I have seen some critical patients being brought back from

the brink of death, and I have also seen those with a high survival chance being swallowed up by death. I know how hardworking every nurse is and how diligently they do their work at the lab. Healthcare professionals put their own lives on hold to treat complete strangers. They sacrifice their personal relationships, hobbies, sleep, and sometimes even their health to ensure that no one suffers on their watch.

To all the healthcare professionals I have had the pleasure of working with in the Cath Lab and to all the healthcare professionals out there, working round the clock to provide care for those who need it, I would just like to say:

"You are all heroes in scrubs who diligently answer the call to serve, care, fight, and save lives. The ones who understand that a patient is more than a person in need; that they require your utmost attention. Being a nurse is more than just an occupation; it is a lifelong commitment to hard work. It is about giving and understanding that this work needs your complete devotion. You leave your personal life behind the hospital's doors and dedicate your life to the betterment of mankind. I salute each and every healthcare professional who lives life on the go, who sometimes neglects their own needs to answer the call and come running to their duties – even if they are in their PJs. You do not get weekends or holidays off, nor do you demand them because you know the weight of the responsibility that rests on your shoulders. This work is not everyone's cup of tea, and not everyone can stomach the things we see and the emotions we experience daily. It takes courage to become a nurse and be dutiful to your responsibilities. To all the healthcare professionals out there, you are the real heroes!"

***

What is time? A number? A specific duration? The Oxford English Dictionary defines time as "*the indefinite continued progress of existence and events in the past, present, and future, regarded as a whole.*" In the Cath lab, though, time is more than just a number or the passage of events.

Our time isn't defined by days, hours, minutes, seconds, or any other mathematical notation. For us, time is defined in terms of muscles – how every infarction becomes irreversible with each passing minute, how just a few moments can mean the difference between life and death. For us, time can pass by in the blink of an eye when we are fighting to prevent damage, or it can stand still when we see a patient's heart rhythm go flat.

Chapter 2
Unforgettable

"Time of death ..."

As a healthcare professional, those are some words you never want to hear, yet they are inevitable. Working in a field that deals with one of the body's most vital organ, the heart, there is always a chance that a case might go awry. Of course, you do your best to ensure that that doesn't happen, but sometimes cases take unexpected turns. While every death you witness hits you hard, perhaps the ones that hit you hardest are those you don't see coming. Those are the cases that are unforgettable because they become imprinted on your mind.

I have witnessed so many instances where everything seemed to be going well, only for a sudden and unexpected complication to arise that completely changed the result. If a patient loses their life because of a wrong decision by the healthcare providers or a delay in treatment, you are wracked with guilt. However, if a patient loses their life because of an unforeseen circumstance, you are left feeling helpless because you know you gave it your all to save the patient, and it still wasn't enough.

Emergencies are part of a nurse's daily life at the Cath lab, and the fight for life and death between a nurse and their patient is a constant and never-ending battle. And during this battle, we are sometimes presented with surprises. For example, we were trying to open up a right coronary artery (RCA) in a patient one time. The patient started to bleed into the pericardium. A pericardiocentesis was attempted to remove the blood building up around the heart, which unfortunately failed. We then started a transfusion, and the surgical team had to operate on the patient immediately to remove a huge blood clot because, unbeknownst to us before the treatment, the patient had a serious condition known as Disseminated Intravascular Coagulation (DIC), in which small blood clots form throughout the bloodstream, blocking blood vessels and hindering the supply of blood to vital organs.

Similarly, there was another case in which a patient coded on the table. CPR was initiated, but the patient, all of a sudden, started coughing up blood. Unfortunately, the patient did not make it, and we later discovered that the patient's pulmonary artery had ruptured during CPR. So, such sudden deaths take a toll on you.

On our end, we make sure to be well-prepared before treating a patient. We have a meticulous procedure in place in the Cath lab because we understand that if a briefing goes wrong, it could result in a death sentence. We diligently follow a systematic approach while assessing the patient. We carefully note their allergies and any medication that can increase their risk of complications from a cardiac catheterization. There is a risk of allergic reaction to the dye used during the catheterization procedure, so being aware of any existing allergies or sensitivity to medication is crucial. For example, is the patient allergic to iodine, shellfish, banana, or latex? Is the patient on certain medications like oral anticoagulants, furosemide, metformin, insulin, Viagra (sildenafil, vardenafil, or tadalafil), Angiotensin-converting enzyme (ACE) inhibitors, angiotensin II receptor blockers, or non-steroidal anti-inflammatory drugs (NSAIDs)? Cardiac catheterization poses a risk of injury to the fetus from radiation exposure that can lead to congenital defects. Hence, it is essential to know if a patient is pregnant.

For this reason, every female patient under 60 or those who still menstruate get a pregnancy test before a cardiac cath procedure. That was the case for a patient who came with her husband to have a left and right heart catheter to rule out congestive heart failure. The patient had a history of Type 2 diabetes, hypertension, hyperlipidemia, and obesity. She also had a new onset of shortness of breath upon minimal exertion and swollen legs.

Prior to the procedure, we did a routine pregnancy test, and to the surprise of everyone, her test came back positive for pregnancy. Lydia was 55 years old, and according to her, she was post-menopausal. I will tell you more about Lydia's story in *Chapter 4* when I talk about congenital defects.

Specific medical conditions can also give rise to certain risks, so we must do our due diligence to ensure that we don't miss out on anything that could harm the patient if ignored.

For patients with some kind of allergy or other medical condition, we pre-medicate them with antihistamines and steroids to prevent adverse reactions during the catheterization or surgery. However, we don't always know about a patient's allergies before we begin the procedure. Although patients with allergies tend to be more aware of their condition and answer all our questions very carefully, many of the surprises we get in the Cath lab also happen to be allergies that the patient either was unaware of themselves or failed to inform us about before the procedure. Therefore, it is essential for patients presenting with heart problems to be aware of any allergies they might have because ignorance or lack of diligent provision of such information can lead to harmful complications, which can even be fatal.

Besides keeping track of a patient's medical history, another critical part of Cath lab professionals' job is distinguishing an electrical issue from a plumbing issue. Blockage of coronary arteries, which can lead to a heart attack, is called a plumbing issue. In contrast, electrical issues refer to heart rhythm problems (heart arrhythmias) in which the electrical signals that coordinate the heart's beats are faulty. The normal heart rate ranges between 60 to 100 beats per minute for healthy adults. If the heartbeat goes below 60 bpm, it is termed bradycardia. If it beats too fast, i.e., higher than 100 bpm, it is called tachycardia. The heart has a natural pacemaker known as the sinoatrial node (SA node), which releases electrical impulses that help the heart pump blood to the body. When this natural pacemaker fails, a small device called a pacemaker is implanted on a temporal or permanent basis, depending on the patient's situation.

A temporary pacemaker is usually used when a patient has a change in heart rate due to a condition or event that can resolve within a short time. These include heart attack, infection, and medication side effects or open-heart surgery. A permanent pacemaker may be implanted if such a heart rate does not resolve over time.

However, when the heart's natural pacemaker is damaged and can no longer generate a normal heartbeat, it is called Sick Sinus Syndrome (SSS). In this case, a patient's heart begins to beat at a remarkably slow rate. Such patients require a permanent pacemaker (PPM) to help the heart beat normally. Although SSS patients might experience dizziness, shortness of breath, or fatigue, they typically do not experience chest pain.

Electrical issues are usually solved with pacemakers or

defibrillators. A pacemaker is a small battery-operated device implanted in the chest that helps control the heartbeat. It signals the heart to beat when it is beating too slow or irregular. On the other hand, a defibrillator is a device that helps to restore a normal heartbeat by sending shock/electric impulses to the heart to correct an arrhythmia.

Cardiac catheterization deals with plumbing issues. It examines the heart's functioning to ensure it is receiving enough blood. There are two types of heart catheterizations, both of which have different purposes.

1. ***Right Heart Catheterization:***

   A right heart catheterization, or pulmonary artery catheterization, is a diagnostic test performed by cardiologists to see how well the heart is pumping blood, i.e., how much blood it pumps per minute, and to measure the blood pressure in the heart and main vessels in the lungs. It is a venous procedure performed by passing the catheter through the veins.

2. ***Left Heart Catheterization:***

   A left heart catheterization or coronary angiography is performed to check for coronary artery disease. It can also be used to diagnose congenital heart disease, cardiomyopathy, heart failure, and heart valve disease. Unlike right heart catheterization, it is an arterial procedure in which the catheter is passed through the artery.

So, what exactly happens during the catheterization process? When a heart attack patient arrives in the Cath lab, we all know our roles and work fast because every second counts when it comes to the heart. Depending on the patient's anatomy and physician's preference, the procedure to stop the heart attack can be done through the wrist or the groin.

In the latter case, the patient's groin is shaved and sterilized with ChlorapPrep, an antiseptic solution. If the physician decides to perform the procedure through the wrist, the wrist is sterilized with ChloraPrep. However, the groin is prepped in either case because physicians sometimes face difficulties in advancing the catheter from the wrist. So, the groin is always ready as a backup to go through with the procedure without wasting time.

While the area for the procedure is being prepared, the patient is hooked to multiple monitoring equipment to monitor their heart rate, blood pressure, oxygen, and EKG. Next, the patient is draped in a sterile fashion from their neck down to their feet to minimize the risk of infection. The patient is then ready for the procedure.

As a Cath lab nurse, I am the patient's advocate. I need to

monitor the patient's vitals and physical condition constantly to ensure all is going well. It is also my responsibility to sedate the patient and administer all the routine medication to make sure that the patient is comfortable and ensure ideal conditions for a successful procedure. Sometimes, a patient's condition can suddenly begin to decline during the procedure, and as a Cath lab nurse, I need to know what medication to administer to resuscitate the patient.

Catheters, wires, and balloons are used during a heart catheterization, and because these are foreign objects, they tend to form clots inside the body. If a clot forms on a catheter or wire in the heart, it can lead to a second heart attack or even travel to the brain and cause a stroke. To avoid such a situation, we give the patients a blood thinner before starting the procedure. Another part of my job as a nurse is to check if the patient has received enough blood-thinning medication before the procedure.

During a heart attack, a slightly invasive procedure to open clogged coronary arteries called Percutaneous Coronary Intervention (PCI) is performed by an interventional cardiologist. The physician starts by inserting an IV called a sheath into the wrist or the groin, and then they advance a catheter through this sheath into the aorta. Once there, the physician directs the catheter toward the opening (Ostia) of the offending coronary artery and injects a dye into it to envision and evaluate the damage done.

Once the dye kicks in and the blockage in the arteries becomes apparent, the physician pushes a thin wire into the catheter and runs it all the way into the artery that caused the heart attack, and skillfully manipulates it through and past the blockage to create a rail for the balloons and stents that are used to clear the blockage. All catheters are inserted and exchanged over this wire. It is like a railway that directs the catheter where to go.

Once this wire rail is in place, the physician then chooses a balloon depending on the size and length of the blocked coronary artery, runs it over the wire, and then inflates it to a specific atmospheric pressure as indicated by the manufacturer of the balloon so that it can squeeze the plaque blocking the coronary artery against the internal wall. This action does two things for the patient; one, it restores blood flow into the coronary artery that caused the heart attack, successfully stopping the heart attack, and two, it creates a nice lumen or space inside the heart vessel or coronary, which is ideal to deploy a stent thereafter. Coronary stents these days are coated with drugs that slow down or completely stop plaque buildup in the coronary artery once it is treated with the stent. And so, it is essential to pre-treat coronary blockage with a balloon to get rid of as much plaque as possible so as not to burden the stent and allow it to work as efficiently as possible.

Once the balloon has squashed as much plaque as it can, its

work is done, and it is removed to prepare for the stent placement. Coronary stents are typically mounted on a balloon and come in various lengths and sizes. The physician decides which one to use by examining different angiogram images taken during the procedure. After deciding on a stent size, the physician inserts the stent the same way as he did the balloon and position it at the site of the blockage. To deploy the stent and attach it to the coronary's internal wall, the physician and his assistant inflate the balloon on which the stent is mounted. The stent opens up like an umbrella and attaches itself to the artery. After that, the balloon is deflated and removed from the body. The deployed stent becomes a permanent implant in the patient's coronary artery.

An angiogram of the stented artery is performed to ensure everything is in place, and if need be, touch-ups can be done with a non-compliant balloon to ensure that the stent is well attached to the artery's wall. If everything looks good, final pictures are taken, and the catheter, wires, and balloon are removed from the body. Lastly, the physician removes the sheath from the inserted area.

If the wrist was used for the procedure, then a unique radial band is used to stop the bleeding once the sheath is removed. This radial band applies pressure to the puncture site and is removed after a clot has formed and there is no more bleeding. However, the groin is at a higher risk of bleeding at the puncture site because it is punctured at the femoral artery, a much bigger artery than the radial one. So, if the groin is used for the procedure, it is important to take necessary precautions when taking out the sheath. The most common method of handling the groin bleed is by applying steady manual pressure at the puncture site for about twenty or thirty minutes or until the bleeding stops after the sheath is removed.

The need for proper handling of the groin area to prevent bleeding complications cannot be over-emphasized. A good grip on the artery must be established when applying manual pressure. Failure to do this can lead to complications such as peritoneal bleed or hematoma. A peritoneal bleed is an internal bleeding in which blood pools or gathers in the lower abdominal cavity. If this complication is not caught on time, the result may be fatal.

Another complication that can arise post-catheterization is a hematoma. A hematoma is a nasty bruise that occurs when blood clots in the tissue underneath the skin around the puncture site. Applying manual pressure to the groin area for such a long time is not only painful and uncomfortable for the patient but also leads to fatigue and finger cramping of the person applying the pressure. Luckily, Cath labs nowadays have closure devices that can be used to seal the puncture wound and stop the bleeding most of the time. Unfortunately, there are also times when a closure device is contraindicated due to a preexisting disease in the common femoral area. In such cases, manual pressure remains the only alternative to stop the bleeding.

Once the bleeding has been stopped, the patient is sent to recovery, where they are monitored closely. An important thing to note is that if the groin was used for access, the patient is required to lay like a log for four to six hours. This is because bending or sitting up causes the patient to generate abdominal pressure, which transmits to the groin and can cause them to spring a leak at the puncture site. Lying flat for four to six hours is uncomfortable for all patients, especially for elderly patients and those with back pain. As a nurse, I ensure my eyes are constantly on my patients while they are recovering. The last thing I want is for a patient to survive a heart attack and die from a bleed under my watch.

It is always exciting for my team and me when a patient undergoes a successful procedure to stop a heart attack. We always hope that the patient doesn't suffer severe or permanent damage to the heart and that they can go on the road to recovery. However, despite our high hopes, not all patients are as lucky, and some suffer a heart attack that causes severe or permanent damage to the heart muscles. For such patients, the road to recovery is arduous and painful with the onset of new cardiac and non-cardiac conditions.

If a heart attack affects a coronary artery that supplies blood to the upper chamber of the heart called the atrium, it can lead to Atrial Fibrillation (A-Fib). This condition involves a quivering or irregular heartbeat instead of a synchronized one, and it can lead to stroke, heart failure, and other heart-related issues. The quivering limits the movement of blood from the atrium to the ventricle and can also lead to the formation of blood clots. According to the CDC, A-fib affects more than 2.7 million adults in the United States and is responsible for more than 150,000 deaths yearly.[1] As Cath lab nurses, we understand the long-term debilitating effects of atrial fibrillation if a patient does not get the appropriate treatment immediately. That is also why we approach and take care of heart patients with such care and urgency.

The treatment of patients with A-fib generally includes blood thinners such as Coumadin and Eliquis, and sometimes even ablation, which involves causing some scarring on the inside of the heart to break up the electrical signals that cause the arrhythmias. Another way to treat A-fib is to use cardiac resynchronization therapy (CRT) to restore a normal heartbeat.

Some heart attacks can also damage one of the two ventricles, the main blood-pumping chambers in the heart. If the damage is not repaired, the patient is at risk of heart failure. Different options for treating a heart attack include medications or implanting a cardiac defibrillator or pacemaker. However, a heart

---

[1] Centers for Disease Control and Prevention

attack is such a multifaceted condition that, despite treatment, it can cause severe heart failure in a patient, leaving only one solution to undo the damage – a heart transplant.

Vice President Dick Cheney, who served under George Bush, knows that all too well. Cheney had his first heart attack at age 37 and would have four more in the next 30 years. The series of heart attacks caused him to suffer from congestive heart failure. After a long battle with the many symptoms associated with the disease, his heart's condition deteriorated to the point where doctors recommended putting in an external pumping device called an LVAD (Left Ventricular Assist Device). However, that was only a temporary solution. Due to the damage that the five heart attacks had inflicted on his heart, the only option left for him to live a decent and comfortable life was a heart transplant.

In July of 2012, 20 months after being on the waiting list, Cheney was matched with a donor and underwent heart transplant surgery. Since then, he hasn't made national news meaning all must be well.

Not all patients are as lucky, though. A heart transplant depends on the availability of a donor and whether the patient matches the donor's heart. Unfortunately, it can take several months up to several years, and as patients wait for a new heart, their conditions severely deteriorate, and many die.

It is not uncommon for heart attacks to cause pulmonary hypertension, which is a condition caused by high blood pressure in the blood vessels that carry blood from the right ventricle to the lungs. The right chambers become overwhelmed and get damaged because of the high pressure, losing the ability to pump blood to the lungs, resulting in right-sided heart failure. Right-sided heart failure causes ascites (fluid buildup in the abdomen), swelling of the extremities, shortness of breath, jugular distention, and irregular heartbeat, to name a few. Severe pulmonary hypertension can also lead to pulmonary valve disease, worsening heart failure.

Pulmonary hypertension can be confirmed by using a stethoscope to detect a murmur or an echocardiogram to check for enlargement of the right ventricle.

Symptoms of pulmonary hypertension are controlled with medications that dilate the pulmonary artery or improve the pumping of the heart and diuretics to remove excess fluid from the body. However, right heart catheterization is the best way to diagnose a patient's pulmonary and other right heart pressures. In cases where heart failure coupled with pulmonary hypertension becomes too advanced, the only option is a heart-lung transplant in which both organs are transplanted.

It is evident just how severe a heart attack can be and the health issues that follow. It is this understanding that has us ready to respond at all times and do whatever it takes to save a patient from the painful outcomes that we witness in the Cath lab every other day.

However, try as I might, I can't save every patient. As a new day dawns, I never know what it might bring; joy from successfully treating a patient or sorrow from losing them. There is one case that I can't seem to get out of my head, and it just goes to show how unpredictable life is and how unpredictable my line of work can be.

A patient named Mr. J arrived early one morning, accompanied by his wife and sister. They were making jokes and laughing as they made their way into his assigned room, and they really looked like one happy family. Mr. J was a middle-aged man, around 59 years old, and weighed 210lbs. He had gone to a cardiologist for a checkup due to recent angina pain. He was then scheduled for a stress test which is used to ensure that the heart is getting enough blood. It can be done mechanically, in which electrodes are placed on the chest, arms, or legs to record the heart's electrical activity while he runs on a treadmill, or chemically, in which chemical agents are injected into the body through the vein to make the heart function as if it were under stress. Mr. J underwent a mechanical stress test, and it was determined that his heart was not getting enough oxygen to perform activities. He was then scheduled for a Left Heart Catheterization (LHC) to determine which vessel was the culprit, and that was the procedure he had appeared for that day.

He smiled as he walked in and handed his registration packet to the pre-op nurse. She took it from him and led him to a room to change into the hospital gown. She also went through the paperwork with him, during which he joked, *"This is like signing my life away."* After everything was in order, she engaged him in conversation and discovered that he was afraid of needles. That didn't come as a surprise to us as most men were, even heavily tattooed ones! However, luckily for both the nurse and Mr. J, she gained access on the first try. Further conversations during preparation revealed that Mr. J owned a pizzeria and was going to hand out coupons to the staff after the procedure.

Shortly after the nurse was done preparing him for the procedure, the Cath lab team arrived to do pre-op teaching for Mr. J about what to expect and also to shave his wrist and groin area. Mr. J was very uncomfortable having a female nurse shave his groin. To make things worse, he was ticklish! Behind the curtains, we could all hear him laughing throughout the process. It wasn't every day that you got to hear a grown man laugh so freely.

After that was done, the family exchanged prayers, hugs, and kisses before Mr. J was wheeled off to the Cath lab. As the stretcher carrying him came in, the other team members greeted him and introduced themselves and the roles they would be playing in the procedure, all to make him relax and be more comfortable. He was transferred from the stretcher onto the procedure table, and the team proceeded to connect him to the monitor and other requisite equipment needed for a successful procedure. His wrist was positioned on the radial board with a brace and sterilized with ChloraPrep, while his groin area was also prepared for backup.

The nurse read a time-out, and then the doctor ordered the administration of some anesthesia to help the patient relax. The method of anesthesia we typically use in the Cath lab is conscious sedation so that the patient can control their airway and also follow instructions. The doctor approached the patient and felt for the radial pulse. He got access with a micropuncture needle and proceeded to insert a wire and then the sheath. The patient was given the radial cocktail and flushed with heparinized saline. Dr. Jay then introduced the catheter into the radial sheath to start shooting pictures of the arteries from different angles. The first angle picture represented was the LAO (left anterior oblique). The first shot looked good, and the LAD (left anterior descending artery) did too.

"How are you doing?" Dr. Jay asked Mr. J.

"I feel hot flushes all over my body; it feels like I just peed myself," he replied. The doctor assured him that it was normal. His vitals looked good on the monitor screen. BP 135/80, P-77, O2-100%, RR-18. The doctor finished taking pictures of the left side

and inserted a wire to remove the catheter while simultaneously reassuring the patient of how well the procedure was going, which it was. Whenever a patient is on the procedure table, the vitals are revisited every 3-5 minutes to help the team keep a close watch on the patient's stability.

Different patients respond to the LHC differently due to different factors, such as allergies, comorbidities, and weight, to name a few. Some become tachycardic, racing toward an SVT with heart rates in the 200s. Adenosine must be within arm's reach in that case to treat fast heart rate. Others become bradycardic, and their heart rates drop to the 30s, sometimes even the 20s. When this happens, atropine is the drug of choice. Other times, the patients are just nervous, and once they find a reassuring hand to squeeze and a voice to talk to, they settle down quite quickly.

Since Mr. J's left side of the heart looked so good, the guess was that either the right side was the culprit or it could be something else entirely. As the next BP was recycling, Mr. J, who seemed to be the life of the room all this time, suddenly became quiet.

"Mr. J, are you okay?" asked the nurse, but no reply. Everyone was watching Mr. J's face. Suddenly, the doctor and other team members glanced at the monitor, and everyone went into a panic. His heart rhythm was progressing from premature ventricular contractions (PVCs) to ventricular tachycardia (VT).

The room that was full of soft music, conversation and laughter just a few minutes ago had now turned into an emergency room.

"Shock him," the doctor ordered. The defibrillator was charged, and the first shock was delivered at 200 joules. The rhythm converted to a sinus rhythm for a moment but almost immediately went back to VT. The second shock was delivered, but no change. Then, all of a sudden, all hell broke loose. CPR was initiated, and the crash cart was broken open for quick access to the required meds. The Code Blue button was pressed, calling for backup, and in no time, the room was filled with different medical specialists, the ER team, the Respiratory team, and the ICU Code team. Epinephrine, bicarb, amiodarone, etc., were administered, and Mr. J was intubated. CPR was long and laborious and went on for more than an hour. Sadly, it was all over when the time of death was called.

This is why this line of work is so unpredictable. Even in seemingly simple cases, anything can go wrong at any moment. The man who had happily come in with his wife and sister, the man who had asked us all to come try his pizza, the man who had been laughing and conversing with us up until his vitals dropped was gone just like that. And that is the sad reality you have to accept when you work at the Cath lab.

Chapter 3
Snatched from the Jaws of Death

Working in a place where you handle an organ as vital and unpredictable as the heart is bound to be stressful. Of course, that doesn't happen all the time, but when it does, the pressure on your shoulders is through the roof. Cath lab professionals are constantly battling with the grim reaper, almost like a tug of war, fighting to keep our patients alive, snatching them from the jaws of death. When we succeed, we pat ourselves on the back for fighting bravely and winning, but then there are times when no matter how hard we try, we lose and witness as our patients slip away.

Moments like these would be enough to break anyone else beyond repair, but not in the Cath lab. Death is a part of our lives, and so we learn ways to cope with the loss of our patients so we can focus on new patients. Still, just because we accept that sometimes death is inevitable, we don't let that keep us from exhausting all our resources and trying until the very end to save a patient.

A 43-year-old gentleman who worked as a soccer coach came in one day with a STEMI. He was having rehearsals with his students in the morning when he started experiencing chest pain.

He ignored it for a while, but when the pain got unbearable, EMS was called, and a STEMI was confirmed. The patient was brought to the hospital, and we started treating him. We discovered through a cardiac catheterization that he had complete total occlusion of the right coronary artery (RCA). We proceeded to do an angioplasty and also a stent placement. After the interventionist deployed the stent, the patient suddenly went into Ventricular Tachycardia (VT). A VT is when the heart, specifically the ventricle, quivers and no blood is pumped to the body, and no blood pressure is witnessed. This means that the oxygenated blood that the body requires to function is not being pumped to the body's vital organs, such as the brain, heart, and kidneys. A VT can occur because of a complication from a heart attack. It can also be life-threatening if it lasts more than a few seconds. That happened with this particular patient, so we shocked him and brought him back to sinus rhythm. We thought we were in the clear because he was stable for the post-procedural routine of holding pressure, cleaning him up, and dressing the insertion site. However, as we got ready to transfer him to ICU for recovery, he suddenly went back to VT rhythm. We shocked him a second time and started him on an amiodarone drip. This antiarrhythmic drug is used to treat or prevent irregular heartbeats. That seemed to work, and we were able to stabilize the patient. We monitored him in the ICU for two days. We then proceeded to put in an Implantable cardioverter defibrillator (ICD)/permanent pacemaker (PPM) to help his heart function normally.

Also, there was a case of a woman with NSTEMI. An NSTEMI stands for Non-ST Elevation Myocardial Infarction and is also a type of heart attack, albeit less severe than a STEMI. While a STEMI is caused by the complete obstruction of the coronary artery, an NSTEMI may have several causes, such as severe narrowing of the coronary artery, atheroma or atheromatous material (accumulation of plaque in the inner layer of the artery wall), blood clot in the lungs, and bruising of the heart muscles. Risk factors include tobacco abuse, high blood pressure or high cholesterol, diabetes, obesity, physical inactivity, etc.

Similarly, a STEMI results in extreme pain or pressure in or around the chest, which can travel to the neck, arms, shoulder, or jaw and can also be accompanied by breathlessness and profuse sweating. An NSTEMI, on the other hand, typically presents as a substernal pain (pain behind or below the sternum) and lasts up to 10 minutes or more. Other symptoms include shortness of breath, dizziness, and nausea. In addition, a STEMI is characterized by an elevated ST wave, progression to Q wave, and complete blockage of the coronary artery on an ECG. An NSTEMI, on the other hand, shows a depressed ST wave or T-wave inversion, no progression to the Q wave, and only partial blockage of the coronary artery. A Non-STEMI isn't as severe as a STEMI because it inflicts less damage on the heart than a STEMI. If I were to differentiate between a STEMI and Non-STEMI in layperson's terms, I would say that a STEMI is breaking news while a non-STEMI is just news. However, NSTEMIs are still heart attacks and need to be treated immediately to prevent them from worsening and possibly becoming life-threatening.

Treatment for NSTEMIs depends on the severity of the NSTEMI, such as how much blockage has occurred. The GRACE risk score determines whether it is low, medium, or high risk. Low-risk patients undergo drug treatment and are given medications such as anticoagulants, beta-blockers, and ACE inhibitors. A percutaneous coronary intervention (PCI) or coronary artery bypass graft (CABG) is usually performed for a medium to high-risk patients to open or bypass the blocked artery.

Coming back to the patient, she had undergone a bypass surgery a year prior and presented with chest pain that day with no ST elevation, but she did have elevated cardiac enzymes. These enzymes are present in the bloodstream in small amounts, but an elevated level suggests that the heart muscle may be injured or may be receiving insufficient oxygen. We also found that she had a lot of comorbidities. Some of these were high blood pressure, diabetes, hyperlipidemia (when the blood has too many fats or lipids like cholesterol and triglycerides), and arthritis, to name a few. She coded three times on the table as the interventional cardiologist worked on her. CPR was initiated, and medications were administered but by the third code, we were sure she wouldn't make it. To our surprise, she survived like a cat with nine lives.

We also have cases where patients react adversely to the sedation and other medication used in the Cath lab. For example, we gave Versed and fentanyl to a patient undergoing a heart catheterization, and he suddenly stopped breathing. We then used reversal agents (Narcan and Romazicon) to bring him back to the baseline.

A patient's death hits us so hard; that's why we try our best to keep it from happening because we form a connection with our patients. When you talk to a patient and learn more about them, they become like family. We genuinely care about the well-being of our patients, both physical and mental, and when they sense that, they open up to us. This also helps us get reliable information that can be helpful in the treatment. For example, many patients do not inform us of their allergies, even if they are aware of them. This can lead to life-threatening situations on the procedure table.

We try to connect with them and show them our concerns, and the more we learn about their stories, the more we empathize with them. Some patients don't like divulging personal information. In contrast, others let you into their personal lives and speak their hearts out, perhaps because they have no one else to talk to or no one else who will listen to their woes. Some of the stories you hear at the Cath lab can break your heart. I have had patients tell me about their life's lowest lows; a broken relationship, a divorce, missing out on a good opportunity, losing custody of children, death of a child or loved one. As these things take such a heavy toll on them, many don't take care of themselves, and that often exacerbates their condition and brings them to us. However, we always enter a conversation with an open mind and never judge our patients for their past or present. Our discussions with our patients also include counseling on lifestyle modification to help them lead better and healthier lifestyles.

Cardiovascular diseases are the leading cause of death worldwide and claim up to 17.9 million lives annually. The primary culprit behind these deaths is coronary artery disease (CAD) which is also the leading cause of heart attacks. Although heart attacks are most commonly caused by CAD, many other causes exist. The most common ones we see in the Cath lab include CAD, drug misuse, especially cocaine, and hypoxia (lack of oxygen in the blood). Besides these, other risk factors include smoking, diabetes, hypertension, obesity, and high cholesterol. Some more risk factors which cannot be helped include old age and heredity.

High cholesterol is a significant risk factor when it comes to cardiovascular disease, which includes abnormal heart rhythms, CAD, heart attack, stroke, etc. There are two main types of blood cholesterol: LDL (low-density lipoprotein), also known as bad cholesterol, and HDL (high-density lipoprotein), also known as good cholesterol. HDL absorbs cholesterol and carries it back to the liver. Higher levels of HDL can help protect against heart disease. LDL is necessary in small amounts as the body uses cholesterol to protect its nerve and also produce hormones. If you produce more cholesterol than the body can use, this excess cholesterol causes atherosclerosis, a process in which cholesterol plaque builds up on the walls of the arteries, including that of the heart. With time, these fatty deposits cause narrowing of the arteries, which leads to a significant decrease in blood flow to vital organs like the heart, brain, and kidneys and sometimes even total occlusion, which can lead to angina or a stroke.

Cardiovascular diseases, including stroke, are the leading cause of death worldwide and the primary cause of death and disability in the United States. A stroke may occur due to a ruptured blood vessel in the brain or blocked vessels or arteries. Blocked or decreased blood and oxygen supply to the brain prevents the brain tissue from getting the required nutrients to function properly. A stroke is a medical emergency, and it is crucial to identify it early on so that complications and damage, such as brain damage and permanent disability, can be minimized. Symptoms of stroke include:

- trouble speaking or comprehending speech;
- sudden paralysis or numbness in the face, arm, or leg, especially on just one side of the body;
- blurred or blackened vision in one or both eyes;
- severe headache;
- loss of balance;
- nausea, vomiting, and dizziness.

There are three main types of strokes, Ischemic stroke, Transient ischemic attack (TIA), and Hemorrhagic stroke. Of these three, ischemic stroke is the most common type of stroke.

It is important to recognize that stroke affects people in many ways, including their personal lives. For example, I cannot forget a patient who had a stroke two years prior and was scheduled for an outpatient heart catheter procedure because his EKG had shown some ischemia on the anterior leads. On the day of the cath, the patient came with someone we assumed was his wife.

As I was doing routine paperwork, which would require the patient to sign a couple of pages, I asked him if his wife could sign his paperwork because of his weakness from the stroke on the right side. He surprised me by saying that the woman in the room was his girlfriend and not his wife. He said ever since he had the stroke, his wife didn't care about him anymore, so he decided to have someone who cared about him. He said the reason his wife still stuck around was because of his money. He told me his wife didn't know about his girlfriend and would like to keep it that way. He then grabbed the paperwork from my hand and signed it with his left hand. I felt sorry for the man and finished the remaining prep work, including getting an IV access that we were going to need for his procedure.

This patient had weakness on his right side from the stroke, so the doctor doing the procedure decided to do the heart catheter through the groin instead of using the right radial on the right hand, which is typically much more comfortable for the patient. The patient was placed on the procedure table, and his groin was prepped and draped for the procedure. After I had performed a time-out to identify the patient and the procedure that we were performing, the doctor started the procedure by numbing the patient's groin with Lidocaine.

Suddenly, the patient started sobbing on the table, and we thought he was in pain. When we asked him if he was okay, he said he was not in pain but proceeded to plead with the doctor to fix him. The doctor replied that he would do his best to fix his heart for him. Then, the patient told the doctor that he was not talking about his heart but his erectile dysfunction problem.

"While you are in the groin, can you find out why my manhood is not working anymore?" he asked tearfully. *"Ever since the stroke, I have lost function there, and it is causing a lot*

of problems in my relationship. I am afraid my new girlfriend will also leave me, just like my wife, who is no longer interested in me. She left the house six months ago and now comes once in a while to see me. I am sure she is with someone else and is only still around because of my money."

The doctor told the patient that he was not an expert in that area, but he was more than willing to refer him to a specialist. The doctor ordered another round of sedation and proceeded with the procedure by putting a sheath in the groin and using the sheath to run a catheter to the heart. He then took pictures of the patient's coronary. The pictures showed a 90% blockage in the patient's coronary artery called the LAD (Left Anterior Descending artery). The doctor fixed it with a stent. The patient was sent to recovery with the sheath still in his groin because his blood was too thin from the blood thinners we had given him during the procedure. The doctor ordered the sheath to be pulled out two hours after the procedure.

Everything was going well in recovery with the patient, and it was time to pull out the sheath from the patient's groin. As described in earlier chapters, pulling an arterial sheath from the groin and holding pressure after a heart catheter is a crucial step because, if not done correctly, the patient can suffer internal bleeding or develop a large painful hematoma on the groin. One of our most experienced Cath lab techs came to pull the sheath. I was standing by as the recovery nurse, watching the patient's vitals and ensuring he was doing okay. The tech pulled out the sheath and started applying pressure to the site. I started the standard 20 minutes timer so he would know when the 20 minutes pressure hold time passed, and then he could check the site to make sure it was not bleeding. I was also checking regularly with the patient to make sure he was doing okay and checking if he needed anything.

Seven minutes into the pressure hold, a woman stormed into the patient's room, flew toward the patient's girlfriend, and started punching her while yelling, *"What are you doing with my husband?!"* When the patient saw this, he jumped from his bed, pulling his IV and wires connecting him to the monitor machine to try and help his girlfriend. In no time, the room looked like a slaughterhouse because of the blood shooting out of the patient's procedure site in the groin. I ran to the phone to call security while the tech tried to get the patient on the floor so he could hold pressure on the groin to stop the bleeding. I returned to check on the patient, who had passed out, likely from the bleeding.

Soon, security arrived in the room and took the two women away. We were able to control the bleeding and stabilize the patient, after which he regained consciousness. The patient was then sent to ICU for further monitoring. We have no idea how the patient's wife found out about the girlfriend or how she found out that the patient was undergoing a procedure there.

This was one of my craziest shifts as a Cath lab nurse and an important reminder of how stroke affects more than just the physical body of the patients we care for; it also affects many other aspects of their personal lives.

Ischemic Stroke:

Ischemic stroke is the most common type; it accounts for 87% of stroke cases and is called brain ischemia or cerebral ischemia. This type of stroke is caused by a blood clot in an artery that supplies blood to the brain. This reduces the flow of oxygen and blood to the brain, and within minutes, the brain cells become damaged and begin to die. If blood circulation is not restored immediately, it can lead to permanent brain damage. It may also be caused by the narrowing of the arteries because of plaque buildup inside the artery walls.

Its symptoms include numbness or weakness of the face, arm, or leg, confusion, blurred vision, trouble walking, dizziness, and a severe headache with no apparent cause. Factors that increase the chances of an ischemic stroke include age over 60, family history, atrial fibrillation (abnormally fast heart rate), smoking, blood clotting problems, injured blood vessels in the neck, and heart valve problems.

Stroke picks its victims with no discrimination, whether rich or poor, highly educated or not, black or white, heavy set or thin-bodied.

During one typical hot Texas summer afternoon, we had a patient that was scheduled to have a leg angiogram done. His name was Mr. Brown, and he had a wound on his right leg caused by PVD (Peripheral Vascular Disease). Mr. Brown had an ultrasound test which showed that the wound in his right leg was due to a blockage to the main blood vessel supplying his right leg called the SFA (Superficial Femoral Artery). In addition, Mr. Brown had a medical history of hepatitis and also a history of IV illicit drug abuse.

During his prep for his procedure, Mr. Brown was urging everyone to hurry up and get his procedure done because he had not had anything to eat and wanted his case done quickly so he could eat. Everyone did their due diligence to get him ready, and we put him on the procedure table. We were now waiting for the doctor to come in so we could start his procedure. Twenty minutes passed with Mr. Brown on the table, but the doctor, for some reason, had not shown up. Finally, the charge nurse called the doctor to find out why he was delayed. When we reached the doctor, we discovered he was stuck on the side of the road because he had a flat tire and was working on replacing it with his spare tire. We felt sorry for him because it was 102 degrees outside, but he said he was almost done and would arrive at the hospital in about 20 minutes.

In the meantime, we were doing everything to keep Mr. Brown pleased because he was not a happy camper due to the delay. However, when we informed him what was going on with his doctor, he was a little more tolerant of the delay. About 25 minutes later, the doctor arrived, looking wiped out from the ordeal he had just gone through in the brutal Texas summer heat. Nevertheless, he was determined to get the procedure started for his patient, who had been waiting for a while. So we finally started Mr. Brown's leg angiogram.

A leg angiogram is where the doctor puts in a sheath in the groin, just like they do during a heart cath. With a leg angiogram, however, the doctor manipulates the catheter toward the leg and shoots dye into the blood vessels in the leg to see if there are any blockages. If there is any blockage, the doctor can use wires and balloons to open it up just like they do in the heart.

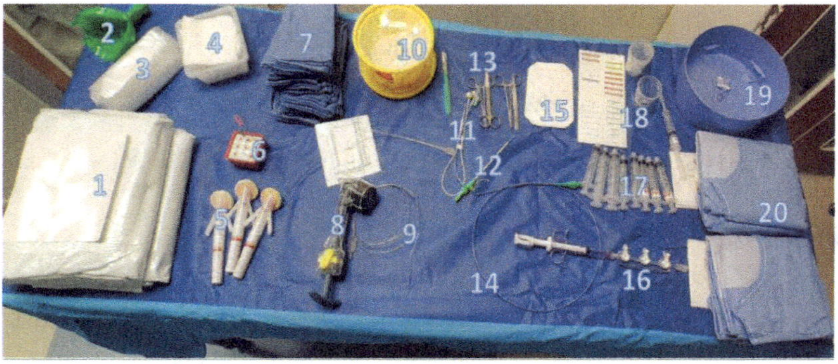

1. Drape, 2. Light cover, 3. Dome cover, 4. Gauze, 5. Chloraprep, 6. Needle holder, 7. Towels, 8. Inflation device, 9. Coronary balloon, 10. Waste container, 11. Guidewire, 12. 6-French sheath, 13. Instruments, 14. Guide catheter, 15. Tegaderm, 16. Manifold, 17. Syringes, 18. Medication cups, 19. Saline bucket, 20. Surgical gowns

So, the procedure was started by injecting Lidocaine into the groin, and the sheath was put in. Then the catheter was inserted, and we started taking pictures of Mr. Brown's right leg. Everything was going well with the procedure when suddenly, the doctor let out a strange cry and fell backward on the scrub tech's table where the used surgical instruments were placed. The doctor had just had a stroke and pricked himself on his left shoulder with an exposed needle on the table that had been used on the patient. We quickly rushed toward the doctor, laid him on the ground, and pulled the needle from his shoulder. His speech was slurred, and he was confused; the left side of his mouth was droopy. We rushed him to our ER, and another doctor came in to finish Mr. Brown's case. It was a rough day for the team because we were very concerned about the doctor. Even if the stroke turned out not to be severe, there was still the issue of whether he got infected from the used needle he had stuck on the shoulder from a patient with a history of hepatitis. Later on, we came to find out that the doctor had a type of stroke called a TIA (Transient Ischemic Attack).

Transient Ischemic Attack (TIA):

A TIA is often referred to as a mini-stroke because it accompanies temporary symptoms associated with a stroke which typically last for a few minutes or hours. TIA is caused by a temporary blockage of blood flow to the brain. Although it may not be an actual stroke, a TIA serves as a warning for a full-blown stroke in the future. People are more likely to ignore a TIA as the symptoms disappear shortly. Still, according to the Centers for Disease Control and Prevention, one-third of people who don't seek treatment for a TIA end up having a stroke within a year.

Symptoms of a mini-stroke include numbness or paralysis in the arm, face, or leg on one side of the body, slurred speech or dysphasia, difficulty understanding others, temporary blindness in one eye, abnormal sense of taste or smell, severe headache, and vertigo. Risk factors include smoking, family history, age, prior TIA, sickle cell disease, high blood pressure or cholesterol, obesity, diabetes, and peripheral artery disease (PAD).

Treatment for a TIA is given based on the severity. Patients with mild cases are prescribed antiplatelet drugs and anticoagulants. Moderate to severe cases in which the carotid artery is severely narrowed may require an endarterectomy to clear the fatty deposits from the arteries. Angioplasty may also be performed in exceptional cases.

Once we got the doctor to the ER, he was sent for a CT scan, and they did a bunch of other tests. The CT scan and blood work confirmed that the doctor had a TIA stroke, and it looked like he would not have any significant effects from the mini-stroke. Of course, blood work was also done to evaluate for hepatitis, as well as the blood work for Mr. Brown to reconfirm his hepatitis status. The good thing was that the doctor was up to date with his hepatitis vaccination. Still, at that point, it was just a long wait for months, including regular tests to see if the doctor had contracted hepatitis from his patient. Two years later, the doctor was still negative for hepatitis and doing well. This event was another instance where I observed the multifaceted effects of stroke beyond the typical physical disability that comes with it. This scenario could have ended badly for the doctor, but he was lucky.

Chapter 4
Miracle in the Cath Lab

"The most incredible thing about miracles is that they happen."

-G.K. Chesterton

In this line of work, we often find ourselves in situations where, despite countless attempts, we are unable to stabilize patients. Of course, we still keep trying, but in times like those, we desperately hope for a miracle to happen. Sometimes, our patients pass away, but there are also times when we witness miracles in the Cath lab.

There have been a couple of times when we have gotten a report on patients with lots of comorbidities - diabetes, heart failure, hypertension, hyperlipidemia, liver failure, end-stage renal disease, stroke, etc. Such patients, have us thinking, *"Where do we start?"* Also, some patients come in with gangrenous wounds, and looking at their condition, we wonder how much life they have left in them, but they surprise us. They go through it and come out stronger. Some come out weaker, but they still survive and keep going. That is a miracle – to beat all odds and continue living.

Sometimes we have patients in bad condition, and we can tell that it will take our all to save that patient. Such a patient is essentially living on assisting machinery and medication like norepinephrine, bicarb, and dopamine, and it's all like a plug. Once that plug is pulled, they are gone.

Of course, pulling the plug is not something we want to do, but there are times when we do have to pull the plug based on family decisions or medical judgment. For instance, sometimes patients become brain-dead, so the doctor, in conjunction with the family, chooses to pull the plug based on medical judgment. Sometimes the patient's family agrees, but there are also times when they refuse to do so because they are not ready to let go of their family member. And so, we see cases like that in the Cath lab too.

One story that always brings a smile to my face is that of a female patient who came to the Cath lab in an unstable condition. Apparently, she had a heart blockage, but before we could even put her on the table, she coded. The first time, she coded while she was being brought up through the elevator, so CPR was initiated. We were able to stabilize her, but as we prepared her for a heart catheterization to open up the block, she coded again. So again, CPR was initiated, and we were pushing in epinephrine, bicarb, and all the good stuff. Finally, however, after prolonged CPR and administering medication but still being unable to get a pulse, the doctor called the time of death.

The patient's family was waiting outside, so we cleaned the body to make it presentable for them. As we were waiting to transport the body, pads were still connected to her chest, and suddenly, she had a pulse. There is a condition known as pulseless electrical activity in which the screen shows some readings despite there not being a pulse. If you touch a patient or move stuff around, you would see pulseless electrical activity on the monitor, so we were all asking, *"Who is touching the patient? Why is there a reading?"* However, we suddenly realized it wasn't pulseless electrical activity; it was an actual pulse! This patient had returned from the land of the dead and had another shot at life.

It was a beautiful moment. All around the lab, you could see emotions ranging from delight to awe. It was indeed a miracle, a work of God. The family had been given the news that the patient had passed away, but 15 minutes later, they were given another piece of news; she had come back to life! It wasn't like we had been pounding on her chest or pushing in medication after the time of death was called, no. This was a miracle, and we couldn't take credit for that. We were delighted for the family that their family member held on to that thin thread of life, and we were happy for ourselves because the Grim Reaper hadn't taken another life from us. The patient is still alive and well, and it just brought us so much joy to know that someone who was pronounced dead moments ago is still living a healthy life.

Patients surviving unfavorable situations aren't the only miracles we witness here in the Cath lab. We often get patients with different anomalies that have you wondering how they have managed to survive all their lives. One anomaly we saw was a patient in his 30s with no right ventricle. The heart has four chambers – two ventricles (right ventricle and left ventricle) and two atria (right atrium and left atrium). How these chambers work is that the superior and inferior vena cava bring deoxygenated blood into the right atrium. From the right atrium, this oxygen-poor blood goes into the right ventricle. The right ventricle pushes this blood to the pulmonary artery, the only artery that carries deoxygenated blood. This blood is carried to the lungs, from where the blood picks up oxygen and is transported to the left atrium. From the left atrium, the now oxygen-rich blood goes to the left ventricle, then the aorta, and is eventually pumped out to the whole body.

This patient came in with a possible STEMI, and as we were trying to put in a temporary pacemaker due to the low heart rate, we made a surprising discovery. The patient had only three chambers instead of four! This condition is also known as Hypoplastic Right Heart Syndrome (HRHS), in which right-sided structures such as the right ventricle or tricuspid valve are either underdeveloped or not formed at all. This patient had never even known that he was missing one-quarter of his heart chambers up until that point. Unfortunately, the patient's heart had overworked itself over the years because of the missing ventricle and was not able to function properly anymore, so he got a permanent pacemaker to help the heart function normally.

Another anomaly that we often see is what we call a myocardial bridge. In this condition, one of the coronary arteries, which are normally on top of the heart muscles, dives into the heart muscle and then comes out again. This causes the coronary to get pinched by the heart muscle with every heartbeat, causing limited blood flow to the heart muscle that is supplied by that coronary artery which can cause chest pain, especially during strenuous activity, leading people to believe that they are having a heart attack.

Myocardial bridges are congenital heart defects in which the heart muscle forms around one of the coronaries during the fetal stage. This condition is present from birth but is harmless for patients with tiny myocardial bridges. For ones with longer bridges, though, they begin to experience symptoms eventually, such as dizziness, shortness of breath, tightness in the chest, pain in legs, fatigue, angina, inability to exercise, and arrhythmia. They can also develop myocardial ischemia, which is a lack of oxygen. When the heart does not get oxygen-rich blood, it infracts.

There are two phases of the cardiac cycle – systole, when the heart contracts and pumps out blood, and diastole when the heart relaxes and is filled with blood. So, an advantage of a myocardial bridge is that during the relaxation phase, the coronary artery is filled with blood and usually does not obstruct the flow of blood to the arteries. The blood level sometimes goes down, though, and produces the symptoms that have been mentioned above.

There are three ways to diagnose myocardial bridge:

1. Cardiac Catheterization:

The best way to diagnose myocardial bridges is through cardiac catheterization. For this condition, we do a left heart cath. When we put in the dye, we do a cardiac catheterization with angiography to measure the blood flow and blood pressure of the heart chambers to check whether the coronary arteries are getting enough blood. If they are, that's good, but if they aren't, we resort to medication to treat it. Patients with myocardial bridges are usually given beta-blockers and calcium channel blockers.

2. Stress Test:

Myocardial bridges can also be discovered through stress tests, which allow doctors to see how well the heart performs during physical activity because, during physical activity, you can tell how much oxygen the heart is getting and how much of it is being utilized. A nuclear stress test can also be used. This test involves a small amount of radioactive material and imaging machinery that takes pictures of the heart, providing information about the chambers of the heart, how well the heart is pumping, and if the heart has any damaged muscles.

3. CT Scan:

CT scans are used to assess the approximate length and depth of the myocardial bridge but are not used as often as the other two methods.

Congenital heart defects (CHDs), such as myocardial bridging, make up a large proportion of the anomalies we see in the Cath lab and are also the most common type of birth defect. These defects can be simple and not cause any problems or require surgery, such as atrial septal defect (hole in the wall between the right atrium and the left atrium) and ventricular septal defect (hole in the wall between the two ventricles). These conditions are not considered as severe because the hole often closes up on its own during infancy or childhood.

A more serious congenital defect is called Truncus Arteriosus. The reason I am focusing on this particular heart defect is that the patient I had mentioned earlier, Lydia, was connected to this condition, so let's get back to her story. Lydia was a 55-year-old patient who found out that she was pregnant when she came to the Cath lab for a routine heart catheter procedure to rule out congestive heart failure due to recent symptoms of shortness of breath and swollen legs. Lydia was shocked by the results, and a repeat test was ordered, including an ultrasound and blood work. The result was the same, and the ultrasound showed that Lydia was four months pregnant.

Needless to say, the procedure was canceled, and Lydia went home with her husband with very tough decisions to make. Everybody in the Cath lab was devastated for the couple because we knew she was going to put her life and that of the baby at risk with the pregnancy because of her age and her health issues. Also, we knew that if the baby was to survive, there was a high risk of deformity and a congenital heart defect.

The couple, on the other hand, was excited about the discovery. They had been trying to have a baby of their own for eighteen years without any luck. According to Lydia, she had once been pregnant at the age of twenty-one. She had a miscarriage and has not been able to conceive since then.

The months preceding the delivery of the baby were a trying time for the couple. Lydia had many health challenges, including preeclampsia, bleeding, and supraventricular tachycardia. At some point, she thought she was going to have another miscarriage. Her Obgyn put her on mandatory bedrest, and she was able to carry the pregnancy to twenty-six weeks of gestation. Lydia gave birth to a three-month premature baby, and it was noticed immediately after birth that there was something wrong with the baby. It was discovered that the baby had a congenital heart defect known as Truncus Arteriosus.

Truncus Arteriosus:

Truncus Arteriosus is a rare defect in which only one blood vessel comes out of the ventricles instead of the normal two (pulmonary artery and aorta). Since there is only one vessel, there is no defined path for the blood. Some of it goes to the lungs and some to the rest of the body. Occasionally, too much blood travels to the lungs, which can cause an excess buildup of fluid, making it difficult to breathe.

If left untreated, it can cause pulmonary hypertension, which occurs due to high blood pressure in the blood vessels to the lungs and can permanently damage the right side of the heart. Babies are usually given medication to strengthen the heart muscle and lower blood pressure. Once the baby is stabilized, corrective surgery is carried out to separate the pulmonary artery from the aorta and to create a connection between the right ventricle and the pulmonary artery. Lydia's baby had to go through multiple surgeries and treatments to correct the defect. She was a beautiful baby who Lydia and her husband named Precious.

So, what causes these congenital defects? The heart begins to form within three weeks of gestation and fully develops by the eighth week. Heart defects can also develop during this time. There can be many risk factors for developing a congenital heart defect, including a family history of heart defects, certain medications, smoking, consuming alcohol, or drug abuse during pregnancy, a viral infection during the first trimester, and diabetes. These factors can affect the formation and growth of a baby's heart and lead to congenital heart defects. Besides these, changes in a baby's genes and chromosomes can also lead to CHDs. For example, approximately 50% of babies born with Down syndrome have some heart defect.[2]

Another anomaly we often see here in the Cath lab, especially in older children and young adults, is the anomalous coronary artery (ACA). These arteries typically have some malformation that is congenital. The anomaly can occur at the origin, location, or some other part of the coronary artery and may affect its size or shape. Anomalous coronary arteries are most often found in patients with some kind of congenital heart diseases, such as transposition of the great arteries (TGA), tetralogy of Fallot (TOF), and pulmonary atresia, to name a few.

ACA presents with different symptoms depending on its

[2] Global Down Syndrome Foundation

severity. For example, babies may experience symptoms such as irritability, sweating, pale skin, trouble breathing, and swelling of the ankles or feet. Older children and adults may experience chest pain, dizziness, fatigue, or they may faint during strenuous exercise.

ACA is a major concern because, often, symptoms do not occur until well into adulthood. Most of the time, we get patients with ACA who do not even know they have it because they have never had symptoms before. As malformed arteries can reduce the amount of oxygen supplied to the heart, they can cause myocardial ischemia and cardiac arrest in older children and adults. Some patients only find out about their condition after suffering cardiac arrest.

The most common type of patients we see with ACA is young athletes and other individuals who partake in strenuous physical activity. Many of them just pass out while playing or doing some other activity and they're gone, just like that. ACA is actually the second leading cause of death in young athletes after cardiac arrest.[3]

Thanks to modern technology, ACA can be diagnosed and treated before it starts showing any symptoms. It is important for parents who notice any symptoms of ACA or any other heart defect to take their child to a pediatric cardiologist. ACA can be

---

[3] Texas Heart Institute

diagnosed through a variety of tests that a cardiologist can order, depending on symptoms.

Treatment for ACA includes a change in lifestyle, medication, percutaneous coronary intervention, or surgery. Medicines usually include beta-blockers, diuretics, and antiarrhythmic medicines. Lifestyle changes involve avoiding certain types of sports and not engaging in strenuous physical activity for long periods. Some types of ACAs can be treated by placing a stent in the malformed artery through cardiac catheterization. If the artery is too severely deformed, then surgery is recommended to correct it.

Besides these many congenital heart diseases, we see several other new things. For example, we all have three major arteries – the right coronary artery, the left anterior descending artery (LAD), and the left circumflex artery. However, I have seen patients who had the right coronary artery coming out from the left side rather than the right. Similarly, I have also seen patients who have extra arteries. For example, instead of one right coronary artery, they have two! And we also see patients who have all the arteries coming out of the left main.

Things like these are not meant to be, and yet they happen. However, the most fascinating part about it all is that the heart has a way of remodeling itself. Even though we see patients who have extra arteries or patients whose arteries are protruding from the wrong places, they still get by just fine. If any one of the three major arteries of a patient doesn't function properly, then we see that the heart beginning to use the other smaller coronary arteries, called the collaterals, to pump blood. If a patient has extra arteries, they all divide the work of supplying oxygen-rich blood to the heart and the body. That just goes to show you how the heart always finds a way. It constructs a new road to ensure that it gets the necessary blood and oxygen. It remodels itself, and that shows you just how amazing God and his creations are.

Chapter 5 Takotsubo

It was one of those days you count the minutes and literally pray that everyone will be fine to enable you to have a quality time of fellowship with your family. It was Thanksgiving, and I was over at my in-laws' house having a good time when the page came through. Upon arrival at the hospital, I discovered that my patient was a beautiful middle-aged woman. We quickly started getting her ready for a heart catheterization to enable us to meet the "door to balloon time."

The standard guideline for STEMI patients to get their culprit artery open is 90 minutes or less to forestall cardiac infracts.

As we transferred her from the stretcher to the procedure table, she asked in a quiet but resolute voice, "*Am I dying*?" The question jolted me, but I smiled and calmly replied, "*No, honey. You will be fine. The doctor just wants to take a look at your heart to find out what's going on with you.*" She smiled cynically and retorted, "*It doesn't matter; I'm better off dead anyways.*" I took her hand in mine and gave it a gentle squeeze. She looked away as a repressed tear snaked its way toward her left ear. I wiped it off and continued to hold onto her hand reassuringly. I could tell that she had raw pain hidden deep in her heart.

We often hear the term "broken heart" when someone goes through a very sad or traumatic experience. Be it a breakup, divorce, loss of a friend or loved one, a missed opportunity, or something else, we are overcome with emotion, and we often describe what we are feeling as having a broken heart. Now, most people out there don't really take this term literally, but what many people might not realize is that extreme sadness can actually lead to a literal "broken" heart. In times of extreme sadness, stress is also inevitable. Going through a painful experience negatively affects the heart and can lead to an acute form of heart failure called Takotsubo Cardiomyopathy (TCM), or "Broken Heart Syndrome." Have you ever seen long-term partners passing within hours or days of each other? It is quite possible that they died of a broken heart. Takotsubo can even affect healthy individuals with no prior heart-related problems.

Takotsubo Cardiomyopathy was first discovered by a Japanese cardiovascular specialist in 1990. It is stress-induced cardiomyopathy. It is a temporary and reversible condition and is often misdiagnosed as a heart attack because it mimics the symptoms of a heart attack. Its main symptoms include sudden chest pain, shortness of breath, and tightness in the chest, while others include nausea, vomiting, and fainting. Patients with Takotsubo often believe that they are having a heart attack until you put them on the table and realize that it is, in fact, broken heart syndrome.

This condition gets its name from the Japanese term for octopus trapping pots (tako tsubo). During Takotsubo Cardiomyopathy, the heart muscle suddenly weakens, and the left ventricle of the heart becomes enlarged and changes shape, resembling an octopus trap. The enlarging of the left ventricle disrupts the heart's normal pumping ability and leads to heart attack-like symptoms. TCM is also known as apical ballooning cardiomyopathy because of the apical ballooning of the tip (apex) of the left ventricle.

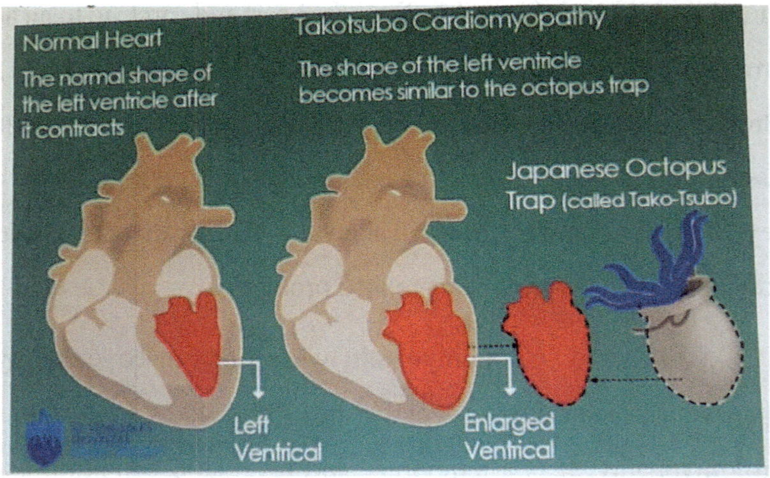

A diagram illustrating Takotsubo cardiomyopathy

Takotsubo usually reverses itself in a few days or weeks, and the patients fully recover. However, for a patient experiencing Takotsubo, especially since it's not very well-known and presents the same way as a heart attack, they understandably freak out. They feel like they cannot breathe and experience severe chest pain. Everything that a heart attack patient feels – Takotsubo patients feel.

What differentiates an actual heart attack from Takotsubo Cardiomyopathy is that in a heart attack, there is a major or complete blockage of coronary arteries, while in Takotsubo, the arteries are not blocked. Instead, only the flow of blood is reduced. Therefore, it does not lead to permanent heart damage either.

The Mayo Clinic defines four conditions for a Takotsubo Cardiomyopathy diagnosis, which are listed below:[4]

1. Transient hypokinesis, dyskinesis, or akinesis of the left ventricular segments with or without apical involvement, and often, but not always, the presence of a stressor.
2. Absence of obstructive coronary disease.
3. EKG abnormalities such as ST-segment elevation and/or T-wave inversion or elevation in troponin.
4. Non-appearance of myocarditis or pheochromocytoma.

When people say, "My heart is broken" or "My heart is breaking," others only take it metaphorically, but here in the Cath lab, we see that actually happening. The heart is really broken and bleeding. This is because, during Takotsubo, the heart muscles are injured, and when that happens, they release troponin. Troponin is a

[4] Mayo Clinic

type of protein found in heart muscles. It is not normally found in the blood, but when the heart muscles are injured, large amounts of troponin are released into the bloodstream. High levels of troponin in the blood indicate a heart attack, so when we conduct a blood test of a Takotsubo patient, we believe they have a heart attack.

Even an ECG or EKG is not enough to diagnose Takotsubo because electrocardiograms for Takotsubo show the same abnormalities as for a heart attack. Therefore, other methods are required to rule out a heart attack. For example, here in the Cath lab, when we get a heart attack patient, we do an ECG and a blood test and diagnose that the patient is suffering a heart attack because the ECG shows ST-segment elevation and the blood test shows abnormal amounts of troponin in the blood. However, it is when we put the patient on the table and do a heart catheterization that we discover the arteries are clear and that only the heart muscle isn't working as it should, meaning the patient is suffering from Takotsubo Cardiomyopathy.

Other methods that doctors may use to diagnose Takotsubo include:

- *Echocardiography:* Sounds waves are used to create moving images of the heart's pumping efficiency.
- *Cardiac MRI:* Generates still and moving pictures of the heart.

- *Ventriculogram:* A dye is injected into the left ventricle, and then x-rays are taken to examine the size and pumping efficiency of the left chamber.

Takotsubo Cardiomyopathy is almost always preceded by an extreme physical or emotional stressor. Physical stressors may include shock, sepsis, seizures, spinal cord injury, drug or alcohol withdrawal, a car accident, and heatstroke. In contrast, emotional and psychological stressors may include the loss of a loved one, breakup, divorce, domestic abuse, loss of custody of a child, or being diagnosed with a serious illness, among others. TCM can also be caused by certain medical procedures and conditions such as colonoscopy, C-section, asthma, blood transfusion, connective tissue disorders, etc. In rare cases, certain medications such as Duloxetine, Epinephrine, and Adderall can cause Takotsubo.

Although these are the most commonly observed stressors for Takotsubo Cardiomyopathy, they can sometimes also occur without any obvious stressors. For example, one in five Takotsubo patients displays no apparent stressors.[5]

More than 89% of TCM cases in the United States occur in post-menopausal women.[6] According to the Takotsubo

---

[5] Pelliccia, F., Kaski, J. C., Crea, F., & Camici, P. G. (2017). Pathophysiology of Takotsubo syndrome. *Circulation*, *135*(24), 2426-2441.

[6] Jain, S. K. A., Larsen, T. R., Souqiyyeh, A., & David, S. W. (2013). Takotsubo

International Registry, 90% of TCM cases across the globe occur in women over 60.[7] A common explanation for this statistic is that estrogen protects women from heart disease, and as estrogen levels decline after menopause, they become more prone to heart-related conditions, including TCM.

The first major case of Takotsubo that I witnessed in the Cath lab was a lady whose husband left her after more than thirty years of marriage. The couple had adopted a son in the early days of their marriage, and for some reason, the son had supported the husband's decision to leave the woman, so not only did she suffer the loss of her husband but also her son. The grief was too much for her to handle, and she experienced Takotsubo Cardiomyopathy.

We also had a widow who had lost her only child and ended up on the table. She thought she could overcome the loss, but she clearly couldn't, as her heart was literally breaking.

Although we mostly come across female Takotsubo patients in the Cath lab, we do get men sometimes too. For example, a male patient came in with Takotsubo. He was a fairly young, middle-aged man in his 40s and appeared healthy too. The stressor for him had been his terminally ill father, and he recently

---

cardiomyopathy: reversible stress-induced cardiac insult-a stress protective mechanism. *American journal of cardiovascular disease*, *3*(1), 53.

[7] Takotsubo International Registry

had to put down his fur baby of fifteen years.

Takotsubo is most typically stress-induced. When we get TCM patients, we ask them if they have experienced any stressful or traumatic events in the recent past, but many of them deny it and tell us no. However, as you try to get past their defenses, they slowly open up, and you find out about all the emotional stuff weighing heavy on them. Even if an event occurred months ago, it can take a toll on a patient's heart and eventually lead to TCM.

Treatment of Takotsubo depends on the seriousness of the symptoms and other factors such as blood pressure. The most common treatment for Takotsubo is through medications that help reduce the stress on the heart and help the muscles recover. Patients are typically administered the same medication as for a heart attack, including ACE inhibitors, beta-blockers, and diuretics. Patients with plaque buildup in the arteries may also be given aspirin and anticoagulants. Patients may also be given anti-anxiety medication to help control stress.

Other activities that patients should engage in on their road to recovery include meditation, yoga, journaling, deep breathing, and other methods and techniques that help them relax and reduce stress.

Most patients fully recover from Takotsubo in a matter of a few days or weeks, while others may take two months. In some cases, however, patients may develop short-term or long-term complications such as low blood pressure, congestive heart failure, arrhythmias, and rupture of the ventricular wall. Death in Takotsubo patients is rare (1% to 2%), but 20%[8] of patients develop complications such as heart failure. Recurrence of Takotsubo is also rarely seen in patients.

Three more cases of Takotsubo that a friend of mine witnessed were of three women, all above 65. The first case was of a 67-year-old woman who presented to the emergency room with chest pain that had developed hours prior while doing yard work. The pain was then followed by shortness of breath. The patient was otherwise healthy and was not on any medication. She did not have a history of drug or alcohol use nor a family history of cardiovascular disorders. The cardiac exam showed no abnormalities, the chest x-ray showed no active pulmonary disease, and the rest of the physical was also unremarkable. When the patient was shifted to the lab for cardiac catheterization, it revealed akinesis of the mid and apical segments of the left ventricle. The patient was diagnosed with Takotsubo Cardiomyopathy and was administered beta-blockers.

The second case was of a 70-year-old female patient who was transferred from a hospital to the Cath lab with a heart attack diagnosis. The patient complained of headache, abdominal pain,

---

[8] Harvard Health School

and shortness of breath. The patient also had a history of coronary artery disease and coronary angioplasty with a stent. The ECG showed ST-elevation, the troponin level was slightly elevated, the angiogram did not show in-stent restenosis, and there was also no myocarditis. The patient checked all four of Mayo Clinic's conditions for a TCM diagnosis and was administered beta-blockers and ACE inhibitors. She showed major improvement after a five-day follow-up.

In the third case, an 81-year-old woman came to the emergency room complaining of shortness of breath when she woke up. She had undergone electrical cardioversion the day prior, and her medical history showed chronic obstructive pulmonary disease, type II diabetes, and hypertension. An echocardiogram showed a left ventricular ejection fraction of 20%, compared to 55% just the day prior. The left ventriculogram also showed ballooning of mid and apical segments of the left ventricle with hyperkinesis, consistent with TCM. Treatment for LV systolic dysfunction was initiated, and excess fluid was controlled with diuretics.

However, none of these cases were triggered by an emotional stressor, unlike the cases I personally witnessed.

***

Of course, there is medication for Takotsubo, but most of the recovery depends on rest and less stress. Therefore, the treatment is more like rehab. We try to talk to patients and make them happy because besides the fatigue, chest pain, and lack of energy patients feel after a Takotsubo occurrence, perhaps the most dangerous aftereffect is depression. During Takotsubo, a patient believes that they are suffering a heart attack and might possibly die or experience permanent heart damage, so they just want to talk about the difficult situation they went through.

Not just Takotsubo patients but all patients recovering from any sickness or surgery want and need that. They just need listening ears who will hear them out. They want you to show them you care; they want to know that there is someone they can connect with, someone who understands what they are going through, and someone who is genuinely interested in their struggles. And so, that is what we do. We lend them an ear, try to be kind and respectful of their condition, and try to connect with them as much as we can. We give their hands a little squeeze and let them know that everything is going to be fine. This is life, after all. There are days when the sun shines and days when it rains, but of course, the sun will come out and shine again eventually after the rain.

The reason we try to empathize with patients is to bridge the gap between them and us. As healthcare providers, we don't even need to try to empathize with our patients; it just happens naturally. We try to put ourselves in their shoes and feel what they are feeling, and although we can't feel what they are going through in its entirety, it still helps us connect with them.

Most of our patients are genuinely grateful for our services. They are grateful to us for listening to them and for genuinely caring about their wellbeing, but then there are also patients who abuse our care and empathy. Such patients just want us at their beck and call, not realizing that there are other patients to tend to or simply not caring. For example, we once had an elderly patient who was very abusive. He would cuss the doctors and the nurses, and he would always be pushing the call button, expecting us to show up in an instant. And it was never even for a serious matter. For instance, I once went to attend to him, and he shouted, "I've been pushing the button for five minutes!" I calmly said, "Sir, you're not the only patient here. Others need to be cared for too." Then I asked him what he needed. "I want some ice in my water." It was always some silly things, but he simply did not care.

I have observed that some patients, especially those who are suffering from some debilitating injury or life-threatening illness or disease, are afraid of their final call and the fear of the inevitable makes them bitter. Such patients then try to rub off on the others around them to ensure that they become bitter too. They have the "If I'm going down, I'm taking others down with me" mentality. This attitude affects those who are responsible for their care. Such patients always answer brashly, as if they are doing you a favor by providing you with information that would help in their treatment. They don't want you to empathize or connect with them. They are fine on their own. Despite the abuse that we regularly endure, we make sure to provide well-rounded care to all our patients, regardless of the way they treat us.

However, such treatment does take a toll on us and leads to what we call "compassion fatigue." Compassion fatigue, also known as second-hand shock or secondary stress reaction, is a condition that is characterized by the emotional, psychological, and physical effects of helping others and is most often seen in healthcare professionals and other individuals working in the helping and healing capacities. Compassion fatigue is not to be mistaken for burnout. Burnout occurs because of the accumulated stress of work, while compassion fatigue occurs due to exposure to traumatic instances. Burnout takes time to develop. On the other hand, compassion fatigue can develop even after the first incident of being exposed to someone else's trauma. Because some patients take advantage of our compassion, we become drained and, as a result, don't have the energy to properly care for the patients who truly need it.

***

Although traumatic experiences can literally break your heart, sometimes positive emotions, such as those evoked during events such as winning a lottery, can do the same. How? Because of "Happy Heart Syndrome." Happy heart syndrome is a rare subcategory of Takotsubo Cardiomyopathy. The International Takotsubo Registry was established at the University Hospital Zurich, Switzerland, in 2011. Researchers analyzed data from 1750[9] heart attack patients with Takotsubo. 485 cases were determined to have been triggered by an emotional stressor. Out of these, 96% (465) cases occurred following a sad event, while 4% (20) occurred after a joyful event such as a birthday party or wedding. These "happy heart" patients also displayed the same conditions as the "broken heart" patients, such as a ballooned left ventricle. However, this is a relatively new concept and requires more research.

All in all, Takotsubo Cardiomyopathy or Takotsubo Syndrome is a common condition that accounts for 2% of all patients and 10% of all female patients presenting with clinical manifestations of Acute Coronary Syndrome (ACS). Although negative emotions are the primary triggers of this condition, rarely, as this chapter has discussed, positive emotions can also lead to Takotsubo.

Although patients cannot differentiate between Takotsubo and an actual heart attack without medical intervention, anyone, even individuals without medical conditions, can experience a very traumatic or very exciting event and so it is important to be aware of the conditions that can and do occur because of emotional stressors.

---

[9] Science Daily

Chapter 6
My Colleague, My Patient

"Please pray for my wife. She has no pulse."

A simple message, yet incomprehensible at first. This was a text message received from a colleague whose wife was also a colleague. Theirs was an inspirational love story. The couple, let's call them Andrew and Julie, met at the Cath lab and fell in love, so it was a marriage made in the lab. It wasn't love at first sight, though, at least not for both of them. Julie was a very experienced charge nurse and a little older than Andrew, who was a cardiology technician. He fell head over heels in love with her, but she wouldn't budge at first, perhaps because she was older and way more experienced in the Cath lab. Andrew genuinely liked Julie, and all of us at the Cath lab could see that. And so, we did what any sensible and supportive colleagues would do; we all pitched in to make it happen.

Sure enough, Julie overcame her reservations about the relationship and began to open up to his advances. Andrew was truly a nice person, and he fell in love with her beauty, intelligence, and many good characteristics. He was also good-looking, very loving, and caring, and he was a great cook – the whole package!

Julie also had a very positive impact on his life. She pushed him to do more certifications, and because of her influence, he gave up on his bad habits. He stopped smoking, drinking, and partying and also started attending Church.

I still remember the day he proposed. It was his birthday; the Cath lab team had booked a restaurant for the celebration, and we all had our parts planned and rehearsed. He proposed to Julie with the Cath lab team and their families present that day. Julie's family didn't live in the US, so he had reached out to them prior to the proposal, and he presented a PowerPoint recording of all of them giving their approval; it was beautiful. We were all very happy for the couple, and everyone, even the little kids who were accompanying their parents, gave Julie flowers. So, in a way, you could say the whole Cath lab made the proposal. They got married, but a few months after the wedding, Julie got into a crisis because she had endometriosis and she had to have surgery. After the surgery, the doctors told her that she couldn't have children as there were a lot of complications.

Despite the sad news, their bond remained the same, and they were happy as ever. A few months down the line, though, she miraculously got pregnant, and we couldn't be happier for the couple. We arranged a baby shower for Julie; décor, food, presents – the whole nine yards, and it was a joyous time.

The day she went in to deliver the baby, we were all waiting outside, calling her husband, guessing whether it was a boy or girl as they were keeping it a surprise. Finally, when we heard the baby's first cry, we all celebrated. However, tragedy struck only two weeks later. That was when we received the text message that turned our world upside down.

Julie had a congenital left ventricular aneurysm. A left ventricular aneurysm forms when a section of the heart muscle in the left ventricle (the chamber of the heart that pumps blood to the body) stretches and becomes very thin. This is usually caused by a heart attack and can leave portions of the heart muscle dead or severely damaged. It can also be congenital, which was the case with Julie. So, she had that condition that she was managing. Over the years, Julie had been under the close supervision of her cardiologist, who had put her on medication and routine imagining to monitor the progression of the disease.

On that fateful day, the couple, still celebrating and trying to navigate their new role as parents, had lunch and decided to rest after being tired from being up for most of the previous night. Julie had complained of chest pain radiating toward the abdominal region. She took some ibuprofen and went to lie down in the bedroom while Andrew stayed in the sitting room to nurse the baby. After feeding the baby, Andrew was changing the baby's diaper when he heard some strange noise from the bedroom. He proceeded to check out what it was, only to discover his wife was having agonal breathing.

Agonal breathing occurs in dying patients who do not receive sufficient oxygen and gasp for air, looking bluish on the face without a pulse. He immediately called 911 and started CPR thereafter. Each compression was torture. He had done CPR at work before but never on a loved one. Although it took EMS 15 minutes to arrive, Andrew felt it took an eternity. Upon arrival, EMS took over compressions and hooked her up to oxygen, EKG, and other necessities. Still without a pulse, they rushed her to the hospital.

She was brought in and hooked up to all the machines and medication, but she was eventually declared brain dead. It was gut-wrenching knowing the finality of a patient being declared brain dead. It was a surreal feeling; one moment, you were treating patients *with* her, and the next, you were treating *her*. We hoped and prayed for a miracle and watched the family members cope with the situation. Sadly, our colleague passed away after that.

It was painful to see such a young, energetic, full of life, and kind woman in that condition. She had a young husband, a newborn baby, and her whole life ahead of her, but that was all gone in the blink of an eye. We had seen her just two weeks prior, celebrating her baby shower with her, so it was tough for the whole team to come to terms with her passing. That was a very challenging time for us all, having to go about our routine without her. Her absence was especially felt in the mornings because it was the time we would gather and be assigned our roles. So now, all of a sudden, there was a vacuum there, and we had to figure out how to fill that hole. It wasn't easy and took a toll on everyone, but we got through it with the love and support of each other because we were a family outside of a family. It was a time of sorrow and grieving, but we held each other's hands and navigated through that ordeal.

I reached out to Julie's friend, who grew up with her and became a nurse together with her. She said, *"Julie was one of the best nurses I've ever known. She was passionate and competent in her work. She inspired a lot of people, including me, and she was a great leader. She made me realize that it's not only about knowledge and skills in the field of nursing but attitude. It was a heartbreaking situation when I heard about what happened to her. I've seen how much she was loved by many, not only her patients and colleagues but everybody. Even in her last breath, she chose to help and to save others' lives by donating her fighter organs to others."*

As I have mentioned before, whenever we get a patient at the Cath lab, they become part of our family. That is because when we meet someone we do not know, we try to develop a bond with them to make them more comfortable. Therefore, we try to connect with them on a familial level, which is why we treat them the same way we would treat a family member and care for them to the best of our abilities. Hence, these patients become part of this self-created family.

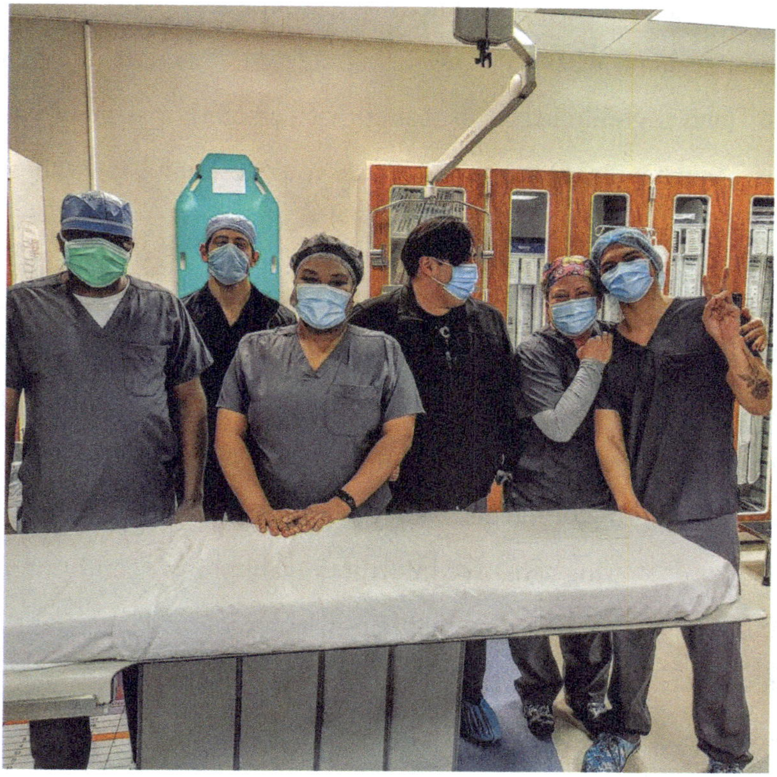

Me and my colleagues in the Cath lab

When we get a new patient, we develop this inner strength, this newfound enthusiasm, that drives us to connect with the patient. We get this adrenaline rush that pushes us forward and makes us want to deliver all that we know. When the patient is a colleague, family member, or somebody we have forged a special bond with, the feelings and emotions are much different. The adrenaline we feel to push ourselves and care for the patient is quickly replaced with a force that sucks the life and strength out of us, leaving us feeling drained and despondent. These feelings intensify tenfold after the prognosis, and you understand what the person is up against. When the reality that you stand a good chance of losing that person dawns upon you, it scares you beyond measure and leaves you questioning everything.

You must be aware that physicians don't usually treat immediate family members. There are many reasons, the biggest one being that their personal feelings might influence their professional medical judgment. Other reasons include feeling uncomfortable in properly examining their family member or the patient being uncomfortable in being examined by a close family member or sharing sensitive information about their condition with them. Of course, that does happen in emergency cases, but these reasons are probably why you can't really treat a family member in the medical field – because of the ties you have with that person.

As a healthcare professional, I don't think we would want to treat a family member even if we had a choice. Having to watch a friend or family member suffer from an illness or disease is one thing but knowing every single detail about their condition is probably worse because although it can give hope in some cases, it can also take it away in others.

Imagine going to battle with an army and losing one of your men along the way. You have to face the battle anyway, but now you have one less man to stand by you and fight. Even one less person can affect the chances of winning the battle, which is what losing a loved one feels like. You have to face a different battle every day, that is life, but you don't have the love and support of that person anymore. It just takes the wind out of your sails sometimes. Losing a loved one is a sickening feeling in your stomach that follows you for most of your life; you can't just get rid of it with the snap of your finger. In times like these, you have to remind yourself of the work you have to do because others need you. However, you can't do that alone. It takes the grace of God to be able to function because nothing stands to reason then. Most of the time, the emotions are just overwhelming.

As much as we want patients that come to the Cath lab to be strangers and develop that special bond with them, that is not always the case. Since we often get emergency cases in the Cath lab, there are times when we have had to treat family members and even colleagues in the Cath lab.

Similarly, we had to deal with the case of a colleague who had an aneurysm. An aneurysm is a bulge that occurs in the walls of an artery when they weaken. There are three main types of aneurysms: cerebral or brain aneurysm (also known as an intracranial aneurysm), abdominal aortic aneurysm, and thoracic aortic aneurysm.

Cerebral/Brain Aneurysm:

Although aneurysms can occur anywhere in the brain, they usually occur in arteries at the base. Brain aneurysms develop when the arterial walls are thin or weaken and cause a ballooning or bulge in the walls of the artery. Most brain aneurysms don't rupture, but if the walls of the arteries become too thin, they can rupture and bleed into the space around the brain. When that happens, it is called a subarachnoid hemorrhage and is a life-threatening condition.

An unruptured brain aneurysm symptoms include headaches, eye pain, vision change, and decreased eye movement. The symptoms of a ruptured brain aneurysm (subarachnoid hemorrhage) include high blood pressure, sudden and very intense headaches, loss of consciousness, leg or back pain, and coma.

Risk factors associated with brain aneurysms include smoking, alcohol consumption, old age, high blood pressure, head injury, family history, and certain conditions such as Ehlers-Danlos Syndrome, Klinefelter Syndrome, Noonan's Syndrome, and tuberous sclerosis.

Brain aneurysms are typically diagnosed through a CT scan, MRI or MRA, or cerebral angiography. Treatment for brain aneurysms includes surgical clipping, endovascular coiling, or artery occlusion and bypass. Other treatments include pain relievers such as Tylenol, calcium channel blockers, and rehabilitative therapy, to name a few.

Abdominal Aortic Aneurysm (AAA):

An Abdominal Aortic Aneurysm is a swelling or ballooning in the aorta. Since the aorta is the largest and main blood vessel that supplies blood from the heart to the rest of the body, a ruptured aneurysm can be fatal if not treated immediately. Just like cerebral aneurysms, aneurysms in the aorta can occur anywhere but are most commonly seen in the part of the aorta that runs through the abdomen (hence the name of this condition).

Symptoms of AAA include stomach pain, lower back pain, and a pulsing sensation in the abdomen. Symptoms of a ruptured abdominal aortic aneurysm include shortness of breath, dizziness, fast heartbeat, and sudden and severe pain in the abdomen. Risk factors for AAA include a family history of AAA, high blood pressure, high cholesterol, and cardiovascular disease such as heart disease.

AAA can be diagnosed through an abdominal ultrasound, abdominal CT scan, or an abdominal MRI. The treatment for AAA depends on the size of the aneurysm. If it is small (between 3 cm to 4.4 cm), lifestyle changes and ultrasound once a year are advised. If it is medium-sized (between 4.5 cm to 5.4 cm), lifestyle changes and ultrasound once every three months is recommended.

However, if the aneurysm is 5.5 cm or more, surgery is performed to keep it from growing and possibly rupturing. Surgery options for AAA include endovascular repair or open abdominal surgery.

Thoracic Aortic Aneurysm (TAA):

This type of aneurysm occurs in the thoracic aorta (the part of the aorta that runs through the chest or thoracic cavity). Thoracic aortic aneurysms are very rare, occurring in 6-10 per 100,000 people.[10]

Symptoms of thoracic aortic aneurysm include chest pain, neck or upper back pain, shortness of breath, cough, and difficulty swallowing. Risk factors include age, tobacco usage, high blood pressure, plaque buildup in the arteries, family history of aortic aneurysms, or Marfan syndrome.

TAA is often identified during routine medical tests such as CT scans, heart ultrasounds, or chest X-rays. Once the possibility is identified, further tests such as an echocardiogram, CT scan, or MRI may be conducted to confirm TAA. Treatment options include surgical repair or removal of the aneurysm or stent placement.

---

[10] https://vascular.org/patient-resources/vascular-conditions/thoracic-aortic-aneurysm

Thoracoabdominal Aortic Aneurysm (TAAA):

If a bulge in the aorta extends from the chest to the abdomen, it is called a thoracoabdominal aortic aneurysm. These aneurysms are the most complex aortic aneurysms because of their location. Its symptoms include constant pain in the abdomen or side of the body, back pain, and a throbbing sensation in the belly. TAAA is most often caused by atherosclerosis, high blood pressure, aortic infection, or trauma from an injury.

An ultrasound, CT scan, or MRI may be used to identify the location and severity of the aneurysm. Treatment options include open surgical repair or endovascular surgery.

So, to sum it all up, we treat all kinds of patients with all kinds of problems and diseases every day, but when it comes to someone we know, our world turns upside down. We have to fight off our emotions and feelings and maintain our composure. Although it is hard, and it takes everything in us, we do keep our composure and go about our day, doing what needs to be done. That is the life of a Cath lab nurse.

Chapter 7
Ignorance Is Risk

As nurses, we develop a bond with our patients when they place their lives in our hands. In my humble opinion, the most sacred object given to us is our being, and the moment we surrender it to someone in respect to make it better than it was, we form an invisible bond with that person. That happens every time a patient is placed in our care, and they hope to be taken care of completely. They expect to be treated fairly, just like any other individual who faces a health emergency. The fact that we deal with people from all backgrounds in the Cath lab has given us a window into experiencing diversity at every corner. We become family with those we treat, and when we see our family not taking proper care of themselves, it breaks our hearts. Indeed, I realize that there are certain things beyond our control. Still, the most devastating thing I regularly witness in the Cath lab is patients suffering through an issue that could easily be corrected and kept under control.

We try our best to keep every single one of the patients in check with their relevant issues and try our level best to advise them accordingly. We make sure that they are not faced with the same perils every time they encounter a health issue which is why we pour our hearts and soul into what we do. The well-being of these patients is our top priority whenever they are in our presence or ask for medical follow-up advice through telephone contact or emails. Even though the human body is a complex creation and many things remain uncertain when it comes to the outcome of certain disease treatments, we make sure that we use every bit of knowledge that we have to bring about the most positive outcomes for our patients. As much as we wish we could know the answer to every problem our family faces, we can only do so much with the tools at our disposal. We can only provide them with the healthcare measures that we are trained for. That is the case we face every single day on the premises of any healthcare facility. Just know that we use every tool in our arsenal so we can expect the best and most favorable outcome for every patient we treat.

So, if you can imagine, the pain is even more remarkable when we see them act in a way that is detrimental or negative to their health.

Often, we are faced with patients who do not take their health seriously. We see them ruin the work we did for them, or they pay even less attention to the measures we have recommended for them to keep their health in check.

I can recall a few cases with patients that were given honest information at every stage when they came into the lab and under my care. These patients showed adamant behavior that could damage their already devastating conditions and simply refused to acknowledge their traits as being the cause of their health conditions worsening day after day.

The first case I wish to share with you is of a woman who came into my care. This woman faced the issue of one foot being shorter than the other. The fact that she knew she had this issue didn't stop her from wrestling with and treating it like a normal thing. Although refusing to feel as though our issues are not as deep as we often feel them is a good thing in some cases, it stops us from overanalyzing and creating an anxious storm up in our minds. However, in the medical world, we must be able to rationalize our health concerns and keep them as honest as we can so we are able to correct them accordingly.

This woman was in love with her obsession with shoes, and she felt the need to wear whatever she wanted without analyzing how her right foot might react to it. Her love of footwear created a cloud of delusion around her eyes in a way that she simply couldn't bring herself to correctly treat her body and not inflict unnecessary pain on it.

On top of the issue with her foot, she was also diabetic, and usually, diabetic patients are advised to keep themselves active to prevent any unnecessary pain that would leave their body suffering. This should be the case for every person, by the way, but the reason it is even more specified for diabetic patients is that the repair time for them after an injury is considerably longer compared to others. In all honesty, the reason why there is such a lack of understanding between the patient and the nurse is that oftentimes the nurses are much more worried about the conditions than the patients are themselves.

The patients, however, stop caring about what happens to them, and they just want the health staff to make their existing problems go away without keeping themselves in check for the future. This means that the care that should be in place but the lack thereof is what is causing the rise of health issues in a lot of people. The medical staff had advised the woman to take better care of her foot the previous time she had come in with issues caused by her shoe fascination. But the heartbreaking point remained that she did not learn from her repeated mistakes. Eventually, she came in with a diabetic wound that would not heal. It started with her great toe sore, which progressively became gangrenous and resulted in osteomyelitis. It got to the point where she eventually came into the hospital with her leg in a condition that only had one outcome of saving her body - her leg had to be amputated. As if the news was not devastating enough, sadness crept in even more when she realized that it could all have been prevented only if she had been more in tune with her body and its issues.

Another case that comes to mind is that of a man who was a chain smoker. Now that could have been an issue in itself, but that wasn't it. This man was facing a condition of coronary artery disease as well. So, all in all, he needed to be a lot more careful about what he was consuming and what monster of a habit was consuming him. This man came to the hospital too many times to count, and still, there was never once a change in his behavior. According to his philosophy, *"Something has to kill a man."*

Every time he came to the hospital for treatment, the healthcare professionals would discuss his failing health and recommend ways to better care for his health. He would simply ask us to fix what we could, and then he would be on his way. There was a time he had a heart attack on a Monday. We worked on him and put a stent on the culprit vessel. He recovered and was discharged on Wednesday. He was back on Friday that same week with another heart attack that had occurred while he was smoking. He was not concerned in the least about the way his body was failing him and that he had made it so. He was merely in the hospital to get fixed for the time being and then kept his routine as a chain smoker.

The disappointment here lies in the fact that these heart-wrenching diseases can be easily prevented with proper care and the right medication before they truly get worse. I am in the field of watching instant results of what can go wrong with your health if you are not careful enough. This is why I am currently writing this book. I want people to be a lot more concerned about how they keep in check of what is good for their bodies and what isn't. The hurt is mutual after years of service in the healthcare industry. Although we won't be in the same physical condition as our patients, once we have properly formed the bond which makes us feel like their family, it resonates to a new level.

In all my years, I have encountered many patients that did not have a single clue as to why they were given a certain item to take better care of their health. As I say this, I can think of one case where, after repeated visits to the doctor, a patient had no clue how to use his glucometer. Being seriously diabetic, he was given a glucometer to help him monitor his blood sugar. He was instructed on how to operate the glucose machine, but he got it all wrong and, most of the time, misinterpreted the results.

According to him, after applying his blood specimen to the test strip, he set it on a stool and waited for the result. Most of the time, the machine only gave an indication of greeting to him with a "HI." However, what he interpreted as a greeting was actually the machine telling him that his blood sugar was very high and that he needed to administer insulin.

Ignorance in terms of health brings with it significant risks.

Sometimes, even if the patients are dying, they are worried about other trivial things. Other things that contribute to bad health include patients not wanting to let go of bad habits, even if they pose risks to their health, such as indecisiveness, sneaking out for a smoke, drinking too much, and not staying hydrated. Not knowing what's bad for you is bad, but knowing what's bad and still doing it is even worse.

This is why the concentration on this chapter is toward making sure that I can make my readers realize how important their health is. We have been given this life as a gift, so wouldn't it be great if we treated it as such? Wouldn't this life be worthwhile if we appreciate the air in our lungs, the food we can eat, the loved ones we cherish, and the beauty of this Earth that our eyes and ears can enjoy?

What I want to make sure is that you, my reader, do not make the same mistakes that many others have made before you. I wish to see people be a lot more vigilant about what their bodies are telling them because, make no mistake, it will. Our bodies are programmed in a way that they can give us indications instantly. They can display signs of discomfort before we can even let our consciousness accept the discomfort. We just have to be brave enough to acknowledge it. I am aware of how difficult it can sometimes be to admit that we have weakened at a given moment.

When we seem not as strong as we usually feel, I can tell you right now that there is bravery in asking for help when you need it. There is bravery in admitting we are not as easy with ourselves as we were at another time. There is bravery in acknowledging hurt and pain. This pain could be mental or physical because, let me tell you, both are valid. Do not concern yourself with what someone has told you to discredit you at any stage of your life. Your pain is valid, no matter how big or how small. It does not make us weak to acknowledge any of it.

Something that I wish to remind you is that even if the person next to you is in a full-body cast, that doesn't mean that your broken arm doesn't hurt. Take this metaphorically or literally, but understand it nonetheless. My goal as a nurse is to keep my patients feeling and looking healthy and to not have them come to me with the same issues again and again. Even though we as nurses are accustomed to seeing people come in again and again with the same kind of problems, the disappointment doesn't fade. I can tell you this much, as many times as we encounter a repeat patient, we never falter with the care that we provide them. Our only intention is to keep them healthy and happy with the care that they receive from us. With the current situation of the world, taking care of our health has never been more crucial. Even a single indication of a cough or sneeze could have the potential to send us into a panic and make us paranoid about whether it might be Covid we could have contracted. Sometimes when people are told to be aware of what their bodies are saying, it can lead to paranoia in folks who have trouble keeping a mental balance of their health and well-being. I understand that it might be difficult to determine whether or not the problem you are facing is enough to consult with the doctors or nurses, but now that we are in the age of accessible healthcare, we should be able to determine that.

It is for certain that when it comes to the topic of affordable healthcare, we have quite a long and winding road to travel. I do understand completely that most citizens in our country are not able to afford a valid or appropriate amount of healthcare. They are not able to afford simple things such as an ambulance or a private room at their local hospitals in cases of labor or surgery recovery. The oldest right in any country is one that is simply called the right to life, and people have been struggling to keep up with the expenses that require a certain cost for living. Keeping our lives up to the mark can cost a pretty penny, to say the least, and most people cannot even begin to spare that penny. Especially in the current climate, with not just our health at risk because of the coronavirus but also our livelihood at risk due to the same virus.

There is always a possibility for change in the high officials keeping their word and making affordable healthcare possible for everyone. But it does seem like a far-fetched idea at this point, doesn't it? It feels as though we keep asking for rain in a drought. For this reason alone, I urge you, my reader, to keep your health above all else. Keep track of what your body needs and what it is telling you to stop doing. Keep your head up high and make sure you do not have to take any serious measures in the future that you could have taken care of today. I urge you to keep yourself educated about the right foods for your body according to what your body indicates. Trust your system, know your system, and understand that *you* owe it to yourself to fight for life. Your doctor can only guide you through the medically right path. You must be the person to show empathy to yourself.

Chapter 8
Shout Out

"In the darkest of times, hope is something we give ourselves. That is the meaning of true inner strength."

– General Iroh

In December 2019, a virus slowly started spreading across the world. Little did we know at the time, it would change life as we know it.

It would be very remiss of me to write this book without dedicating an entire chapter to nurses working during the ongoing COVID-19 pandemic. They are the essence of all that is good about humanity, and they are the real warriors of this pandemic. The spread of COVID brought with it the closure of many industries. Schools, offices, restaurants, stores, everything was closed. However, the one industry that remained open 24/7 and the people who were on duty throughout this ordeal were healthcare professionals. When everyone stayed in their homes, nurses stepped up and stepped in. Despite knowing the dangers of handling patients with the virus, they put their lives on the line in order to save others. Even though they didn't have a choice in the matter, even if they did, they wouldn't have done anything differently; that's just how nurses are. They do what they do. They are warriors full of resilience and true compassion. I truly commend and applaud all the healthcare professionals around the world who helped fight against this deadly virus; those who lost their lives during this fight, those who sacrificed their health for the health of others, and those who are still standing on their feet. Kudos to every single one of you!

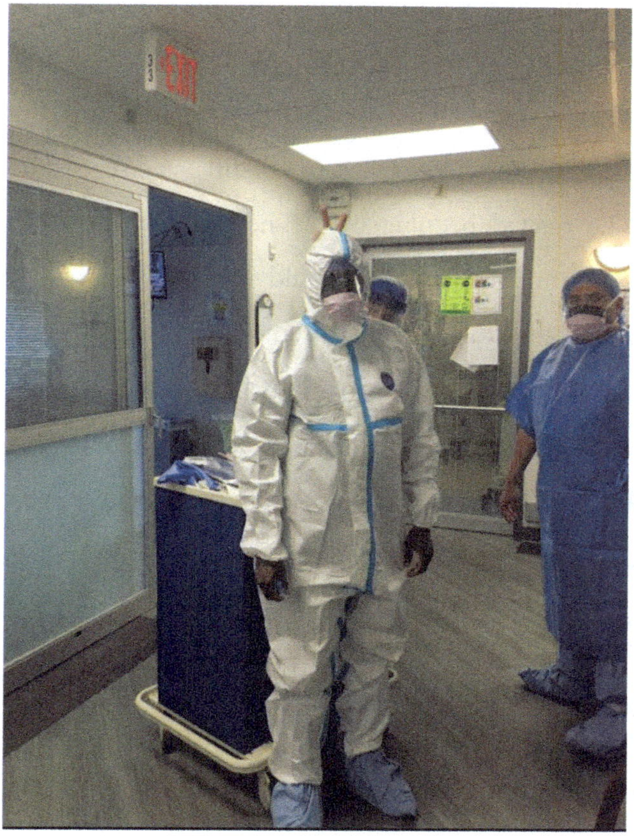

A healthcare professional in PPE (Personal Protective Equipment) during COVID-19

Although the situation has gotten much better now, I know firsthand what it was like for healthcare professionals in the beginning. As COVID approached, the responsibilities I usually had at the Cath lab were soon going to become much more than I could have ever anticipated. As soon as COVID hit, I was no longer a nurse in the Cath lab. I was now also an ER nurse and a radiology nurse. I was helping out in the ICU and wherever else I was needed. I can't even put into words what the rush hour chaos of that time was like. I now have a little less intensity in my soul to tell you how the time flowed within those walls of sanitized interior blended with adrenaline. It was almost like synesthesia for us when we stood still for a second to catch our breath. The rushed beeping of the heart monitors slowly became embedded in our eardrums. We could smell the large range of scents mixing in the air like a cocktail of emotions running high, the scents of medication, and the noise of various IV stands being run across the premises. It was a true experience met with the realization that things had gotten to a phase of extreme surrealness. We were entering an era of caution in our lives that would not leave anything unchanged.

When COVID was at an all-time high, the heroism I witnessed within those walls while going through the motions was of a nature I had never dealt with before. I had seen my fellow nurses and our head doctors perform amazing miracles before. I had seen them bring life to fading souls and give grace to the unsavable ones before, but what I witnessed then was nothing short of a series of heroic acts of magic. It was as if the strength that magically appeared in my fellow frontline professionals was that of war heroes you only read about in history books or saw in the middle of a battlefield. They were indeed heroes, fighting a grave battle. The intense feeling of acting lightning fast to save as many lives as possible that were coming in record time was the crux of all that we had sworn to do for the good of humanity. All our abilities were being used at once, for multiple souls at a time.

Initially, there was a shortage of safety equipment such as PPEs (Personal Protective Equipment), so you would find us, nurses, sharing the equipment or recycling it. So, not only were we working longer shifts and engaging in experimental treatments, but we were also very much exposed to the virus ourselves because the protective gear was limited. I remember so many patients were being rushed into the hospital, so much so that we were treating more people than we had the capacity for. It was all too much for nurses. In addition, there were many patients who had comorbidities other than COVID, some were obese, and you had to turn these patients to treat them and just take care of them while also taking care of yourself. Still, that didn't stop nurses from doing what was required of them. I don't know how we did it, but we got it done.

I believe the terror of this disease was the spreading force of it. The speed at which this virus spread was much greater than the intensity with which it attacked the human body and its effects on it afterward. That's not to say that the virus was not harmful, as it took millions of lives across the globe, but what I am trying to say is that for many patients, their fear of the virus was more potent than its symptoms. For example, I had a patient who asked me, *"So, do I have two weeks to live?"* because they thought everyone with COVID was bound to die. For many patients, COVID-19 was nothing short of a death sentence. They thought that was it for them. They feared it so much, especially because of the thought of not being able to breathe, being put on BiPap, or just feeling their life slipping away. There was just so much fear all around.

Perhaps the most heartbreaking thing that happened during COVID was affected patients being separated from their families. Many of them did not make it out alive, and they passed away, fighting all alone. It's saddening to even think about it, and I can't imagine what it must have been like to watch your loved ones deal with the horrific pain and anguish of this deadly virus alone because you weren't allowed to be with them, fearing the spread of the virus. I saw the weight manifest on the shoulders of my fellow nurses, who bore it all through the pandemic. I also saw this weight in the eyes of the loved ones who were not only forced to maintain distance from their loved ones in their final days but then had to bury them, covered in protective attire. Not only that, they had to maintain their distance from the body.

All hospitals around the world received a huge influx of patients with and without COVID. During this time, not only did nurses have to step up in terms of their services, but they also had to step up and step in as substitute family members for their patients. My comrades and I formed a connection with each of the souls that entered this circle of chaos. The first and foremost thing we had to do was to help our patients overcome their fears of the virus. In the golden words of Nelson Mandela, "*I learned that courage was not the absence of fear, but the triumph over it. The brave man is not he who does not feel afraid, but he who conquers that fear.*" That is what we tried to do with our patients; we tried to help them let go of their fears.

Some patients with COVID-19 would display severe symptoms. However, even those with mild symptoms would be freaking out because they thought that it would surely kill them. So, we had to provide them with support and assure them that they would be okay. We tried to put a smile on their faces. We told them that they would be okay, that they were more than COVID and would come out victorious on the other side.

Besides the fear, we also had to help our patients overcome the loneliness they faced in isolation. In the absence of their family, most patients were stuck in isolation and the burden of going through the recovery stages by themselves. The pressure itself was crushing. Most of the patients felt like this diagnosis was a death sentence, but even for the ones that were given reassurance to a certain extent that they would be able to recover, it was still an uphill battle. The family members of these patients could not simply come to see if their beloved spouse, mother, father, son, or daughter was in a better condition or not. In these cases, we were the ones holding their hand, giving them as much reassurance as we could possibly muster.

There were instances where many of my patients felt like the world had deserted them, which, of course, was not true, but the atmosphere of life at that stage was such that none of them could believe in the future. This is where empathy for them came in tenfold. We became their surrogate family in a strange but, at the same time, very authentic way. The essence of our job, which is to provide healthcare to those in a stage of suffering, multiplied in a way we had never thought possible. Being a Cath lab nurse was no longer my one and only point of responsibility. I was now also a companion for my patients.

I feel that the fear and isolation took a bigger toll on COVID patients than COVID itself, and at times like those, we were with the patients. We were with them every step of the way, holding their hands and giving them a reassuring pat on the back. Even in their last moments, we held their hands as they made their final transition. We made sure to give our patients the best care that we could, considering the circumstances, and ensured that they didn't die alone.

I couldn't bear to imagine what I would have done if I were in my patients' spot. I was traveling within a different boat alongside my fellow nurses while my patients were in another, but I do believe the body of water was the same. This ocean of chaos we all seemed to be part of was making its own valiant efforts to swallow us whole. The love that my fellow nurses shared with the patients and the bravery that our patients exhibited during these trying times truly overwhelmed me.

The first wave of COVID turned us into the medical soldiers you see before you today. The sacrifices we made in order to care for those affected by the virus cannot be filled into the limited pages of this book. The sheer magnitude of missed birthdays, anniversaries, quality time with family, and bedtime tuck-ins cannot be measured by any number. Sometimes, we would not go home for days because there were just so many patients to look after. Other times, we would only go home for a couple of hours of shut-eye and then rush back to the hospital. Many of my fellow nurses have children of their own, but we all had to abandon our families temporarily so that we could fulfill the oath we took when becoming nurses.

The bravery and determination of my nurse brothers and

sisters that were previously overlooked by the masses changed overnight with the effects of the current pandemic. I guess you can call this a silver lining amidst this dark cloud of chaos and despair. As human beings, that is all we can do at the end of the day, isn't it? Look for the silver lining. Since the start of this pandemic, the baseline of what I have learned so far is that we are nowhere without hope. The words of Andy Dufresne resonate with me when I think of the sacrifices we healthcare professionals have made amidst the pandemic. *"Hope is a good thing, maybe the best of things, and no good thing ever dies."*

Our patients got a much-needed reprieve when the hospital allowed us to set up iPads and other devices for them to FaceTime with their families. This had a great impact on our patients because even though their friends and family couldn't be with them in person, they could at least still see them and talk to them virtually. I noticed how having their families interact with them helped many patients recover quickly.

As I mentioned before, despite being a Cath lab nurse, I was playing many different roles when the pandemic was at its worst, and the same goes for many other nurses. We were all doing things that did not fall under our domain simply because we didn't have enough people to do them. The Cath lab really stepped up during that time. We all came together and supported the other teams because ERs were flooded, with people coming in and going out and being transferred; it was all utter chaos. Still, we made it out because we had each other's backs.

Keeping our heads up high seemed like an uphill battle in these times because it felt like it would never end. However, the strongest parts of our beings held onto hope; hope that it would end, hope that everything would go back to normal. Not sooner, perhaps, but definitely later. Hope is what got us through. These were the darkest times for me and the nurses of my generation. The more I try to put into words the amount of physical and emotional labor we went through, it never seems enough. I am a small part of the mass of frontline healthcare professionals and the first responders of this pandemic, but the legitimate appreciation I feel for every single person is what I hope to convey through this book.

I would also like to commend and share some words of appreciation for the new nurses who are stepping into the nursing profession. This is a very trying time to be a nurse, and learning to navigate through the current challenges, even more so. So, I salute the new nurses who, despite the circumstances, are willing to step into this field to serve others.

Made in the USA
Monee, IL
03 November 2026

67388675R00066